Five Centuries of
VETERINARY MEDICINE

Five Centuries of VETERINARY MEDICINE

A SHORT-TITLE CATALOG *of the* WASHINGTON STATE UNIVERSITY VETERINARY HISTORY COLLECTION

COMPILED, WITH ANNOTATIONS AND INDEXING,
BY J. FRED SMITHCORS (DVM, PHD)
AND ANN SMITHCORS (RN)

FOREWORD BY JOHN F. GUIDO

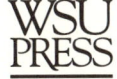

Washington State University Press
PO Box 645910
Pullman, WA 99164-5910
(800) 354-7360

Washington State University Press, Pullman, WA 99164-5910
© 1997 by the Board of Regents of Washington State University
All rights reserved
First printing 1997

Printed and bound in the United States of America on pH neutral, acid-free paper. No part of this book may be reproduced or transmitted in any form or by any means, electronic or mechanical, including recording, photocopying, or by any information storage or retrieval system, without permission in writing from the publisher.

Library of Congress Cataloging-in-Publication Data
Washington State University. Veterinary History Collection
    Five centuries of veterinary medicine : a short-title catalog of the Washington State University Veterinary History Collection / compiled, with annotations and indexing, by J. Fred Smithcors and Ann Smithcors ; foreword by John Guido.
       p.   cm.
    Includes index.
    ISBN 0-87422-141-2 (pbk. : alk. paper).—ISBN 0-87422-142-0 (hard : alk. paper)
    1. Veterinary medicine—Washington—Pullman—Bibliography—Catalogs. 2. Washington State University. Veterinary Medicine/Pharmacy Library—Catalogs. 3. Washington State University. Veterinary History Collection—Catalogs. I. Smithcors, J. F. II. Smithcors, Ann, 1934- . III. Title.
Z6674.W37   1997
[SF607]
016.636089—dc20   96-35493
                                                                                 CIP

Contents

Foreword, by John F. Guido .... vii-ix
Preface, by J. Fred Smithcors .... xi-xii
Catalog—Five Centuries of Veterinary Medicine 1-126
Appendix 127-132
Appendix Index 133-134
Index 135-145

Foreword

The Smithcors Collection of Veterinary History was formed over a period of 35 years by J.F. Smithcors, DVM, PhD, who developed the first course in veterinary history (1955) to be taught at any school or college of veterinary medicine in the United States (Michigan State University). The author of three major works in the field of veterinary history—*Evolution of the veterinary art*, 1957; *The American veterinary profession*, 1963; and *The veterinarian in America, 1625-1975*, 1975, and more than 150 journal articles, papers, and book chapters—he is regarded by his peers as the "dean of American veterinary historians."

Smithcors began donating the collection—then comprising some 1,200 printed books and pamphlets, as well as manuscripts and ephemera, dating from the sixteenth to the twentieth century—to Washington State University in 1978. Three years later, in 1981, he established the Marty Smithcors Memorial Endowment in honor of his first wife, Marty, who died that same year. A portion of the income from the fund is used to support the collection.

The Veterinary History Collection at WSU now consists of almost 1,900 items—monographs, journals, pamphlets, manuscripts, archival records, and ephemera, more than 1,800 of which are described in this catalog—and is growing. There are nine items from the sixteenth century described here, 22 from the seventeenth, 124 from the eighteenth, and more than 1,100 from the nineteenth century, including journals.

The great majority of the works are in English, published in Britain and the United States, but some of the more important foreign-language works are also present: early French and Italian works on the horse—Grisone's *Ordini di cavalcare*, 1553 (660); La Fosse's monumental work on equine anatomy and disease, *Cours d'hippiatrique*, 1772 (868); Ruini's *Anatomia del cavallo*, 1707 (1255); Rusius's *Opera de l'arte del malscalcio*, 1543 (1264); three editions of Solleysel's *Le parfait mareschal*, 1682, 1702, 1711 (1351-1353), as well as the German Seuter's *Ein vast schones und nutzliches Beuch*, 1588 (1296).

As might be expected, British works are well represented, including a number of rarities. Andrew Snape's *The anatomy of an horse*, 1683, from the seventeenth century is present (1349), as is George Stubb's Herculean *The anatomy of the horse* from the eighteenth, 1766 (1400), "the first original work on equine anatomy after Ruini." The immensely popular works of Gervase Markham, also from the seventeenth century, are included (978-984), perhaps the most prominent being a copy of the scarce first edition of his *Markhams maister-peece*, 1610 (982), which eventually went through 21 editions.

One of the strengths of the collection at Washington State University, however, lies in the large number of American works present. Again, as might be expected, many of the early works were derivative. Two of the earliest American imprints in the collection, editions of *The citizen and countryman's experienced farrier*, 1764, 1797 (985, 986), in fact are based on *Markhams maister-peece*.

On the other hand, Paul Jewett's *The New-England farrier* (and variations thereof) is present in five editions—1821, 1822, 1826, 1828, 1835 (809-813). As Smithcors notes in his annotation (809) the first edition of Jewett's work, published in the eighteenth century (1795), was perhaps the first work "native to the United States." Richard Mason's *The gentleman's new pocket farrier* (and variations thereof), present in nine nineteenth-century editions beginning with that of 1825 (992-1000), could be said to have carried on the *new tradition* established by Jewett.

While these early American works might impart a glimpse of the future and the distinctly national orientation the development of the collection would take, English imprints continue to hold their own with American throughout the early decades of the nineteenth century. It is not until after the middle of the century and more especially during the last quarter and into the twentieth century—when American veterinary medicine became less derivative, came to recognize and accept the importance of science and its application to medicine, and took on more of the standards associated with a profession—that the collection reflects a geographic shift in orientation quantitatively.

This geographic shift from the "Old World" to the "New" is perhaps best illustrated by the large number of works in the collection of the pioneering American George Dadd, some 30 in number (379-408), which appeared between 1850 and 1915. The publications of another American, James Law, appearing between 1876 and 1912, occupy 13 entries in the catalog. American works predominate in the twentieth century.

Chronologically the collection spans five centuries, from the sixteenth through the twentieth century. Because of the historical nature of the collection, with some few exceptions, works published after 1950 are not included. The current requirements of practicing veterinarians, as well as those of students, faculty, and researchers in the College of Veterinary Medicine, are ably addressed by my colleague Vicki Croft and her staff in Washington State University's Veterinary Medicine/Pharmacy Library.

The collection, while historical in composition, is not meant to be principally of antiquarian interest. While serving to complement the *current* collection maintained by the Veterinary Medicine/Pharmacy Library, the Veterinary History Collection also supports research in contemporary and related fields. The large number of entries devoted to "Animal Welfare" in the main body of the catalog graphically illustrates these functions, as do the archival records of the Association for Women Veterinarians (Appendix A007), and those of the Delta Society, "an international educational, research and service resource on the relationships between people, animals, and the environment," whose records, unfortunately, were accessioned into the collection too late to be included in this catalog.

The contents of the catalog, both the main section and the appendix, are in an alphabetical author-title-subject arrangement. The index for the main body of the catalog is a subject index exclusively; that for the appendix, while predominantly a subject index, also contains proper names as authors. The cut-off date for inclusion in the catalog was December 1993. Subsequent additions to the collection may be accessed by means of the WSU Libraries' on-line catalog. Since the primary audience for the catalog was not expected to be collectors or bibliophiles, elaborate bibliographic descriptions have been forsaken in favor of brevity.

We are most grateful to J.F. Smithcors and his wife Ann, not only for his efforts in building the collection and donating it to Washington State University, but for their continuing interest and support in helping us develop it, and for their commitment, both intellectually and financially, to the preparation and publication of this catalog. To my colleagues in Manuscripts, Archives and Special Collections (identified elsewhere by Smithcors in his Preface) who labored long and hard in assisting the Smithcors over a period of several years, a special note of thanks. Last, but certainly not least, I must also extend my genuine thanks and appreciation to Leo K. Bustad, Dean Emeritus of the College of Veterinary Medicine, for his early enthusiasm and encouragement in helping to make the Veterinary History Collection a reality at Washington State University.

John F. Guido, Head
Manuscripts, Archives and Special Collections
Washington State University Libraries

Preface

This catalog is designed to increase the accessibility and usefulness of the Washington State University Veterinary History Collection, especially for persons having little familiarity with the early veterinary literature. The entries are based on printouts of individual and collated items as catalogued by the WSU Libraries staff, many of which were in short-title form. To save space, some of these have been further shortened to an extent that does not interfere with the intended sense of the title.

Of the more than 1,800 titles dating from 1550 to 1990, some 1,200 were in the collection I gathered while a staff member at Michigan State University, in conjunction with an extensive program of teaching, research and writing in this area. These items are identified by a § following the entry.

Anonymous works are grouped by subject matter, *e.g.*, Almanacs, Animal disease, etc. Some authored entries are also grouped to facilitate access to them, *e.g.*, Animal welfare, Dictionaries, etc. Grouped entries are as follows:

Almanacs	US Army Veterinary Service
Animal disease	US Dept of Agriculture
Animal welfare	USDA Bureau of Animal Husbandry
Catalogs	Veterinary associations
Dictionaries	Veterinary colleges
Great Britain	Veterinary history
Horses	Veterinary periodicals

The annotations are meant to give only a brief indication of the content and/or relative value of that work. In the latter regard they are subjective, and a characterization as retrograde or worthless at the time of publishing does not mean the work has no value in such a collection. Thus the writings of Gervase Markham, wretched as they were even in the 17th century, nevertheless constitute an important chapter in the history of veterinary medicine—which in Britain and to some extent in America would have been different had he not published these works. The Smith whose commentary is referred to in some annotations is Sir Frederick Smith, author of *The early history of veterinary literature* (item 1328).

The Index affords ready access to some 400 subjects likely to be of interest to persons delving into the early literature. Many of these works, of course, contain a multitude of other topics, which will become apparent when any of them are handled. For anyone wanting a general overview of veterinary history, the entry for History gives 14 such works under the subentry Vet med, and there are 46 subentries for more specialized topics. For works with several editions, usually only one early edition is indexed; it may be fruitful to look into later editions, although in many instances these are little more than reprints. Some of the more important sources for most topics are given in **bold face**, and an asterisk (*) indicates works published before 1800, or those dealing largely with this period. Where appropriate, species are indicated by a letter code preceding the item number.

The Appendix (separately indexed) is devoted to non-book materials in the collection. It describes manuscripts and archival collections, graphics, reprints, unpublished materials, and ephemera. Because of the nature of the material, it has been arranged more along archival principles than book or monographic cataloging principles. Catalog numbers have not been assigned to each item, as in the main (first) part of the catalog. Rather, catalog numbers have been largely reserved for clusters of documents, either those having a common denominator in terms of subject matter, or having been created by a single individual or organization.

Special mention is due my wife Ann, whose enthusiastic and at times total attention to this subject has made her not only highly knowledgeable on the matter but a worthy coequal in production of this catalog. Neither of us is a bibliographer, and we wish to acknowledge the indispensable groundwork done by various WSU Library workers and, especially, the guidance of John Guido, Laila Miletic-Vejzovic, Julia King, and Leila Luedeking. We also wish to thank the Washington State University Press for its meticulous work in producing so handsome a volume.

J. Fred Smithcors
Santa Barbara, California

Catalog
Five Centuries of Veterinary Medicine

001. (ACTINOMYCOSIS). Illinois Board of Livestock Commissioners. Special report...on actinomycosis. **1890**. Springfield, IL: Springfield Printing Co. 37 pp.
   An outbreak with human involvement.

002. **ADAMS, Arthur** (ed). The history of the Worshipful Company of Blacksmiths from early times until the year 1785... **1951**. London: Sylvan Press. 207 pp. §
   With reproductions from original books.

003. **AGASSIZ, Louis** (1807-1883). Histoire naturelle des poissons d'eau douce de l'Europe centrale. **1839**. Neuchatel: The author. 326 pp.
   Natural history of European fishes.

004. **AGRIPPA von NETTESHEIM** (1486?-1535). Paradoxe sur l'incertitude, vanite, et abus des sciences...de choses contre la commune opinion. **1617**. [s.l. s.n.] 306 pp. §
   Speaks highly of veterinarians and scorns physicians who disdain animal medicine. (see Smith, vol l, p 135)

005. **(ALBERTUS MAGNUS)** (1193?-1280). Albertus Magnus: being the approved, verified, sympathetic ad natural Egyptian secrets, or, white and black magic for man and beast... **ca 1900**. [s.l. s.n.] 208 pp. §
   A late edition of these magical cures.

006. **ALBRECHTSEN, J.** The sterility of cows, its causes and treatment. Trans by H. Wehrbein. **1917**. Chicago: Alex Eger. 98 pp.
   Results of a noted Danish specialist.

007. **(ALDROVANDI, Ulisse)** (1522-1605). Aldrovandi on chickens. The ornithology of Ulisse Aldrovandi (1600) volume II, book XIV. Trans, with notes, by L.R. Lind. **1963**. Norman: Univ of Oklahoma Press. 36 + 447 pp. §
   A modern version of a classic, including uses of chicken parts in medicine.

008. **ALEXANDER, Alexander Septimus** (1860-). Udder diseases of the cow, and related subjects. **1929**. Boston: R.G. Badger. 215 pp.
   Diagnosis and treatment of common diseases.

009. **ALLEN, Joseph Alexander** (1886-); **McLURE, W.C.S.** Theory and practice of fox ranching. **1926**. Charlottetown, Can: Irwin Printing Co. 242 pp.
   Management and diseases of foxes.

010. **ALLEN, Lewis Falley** (1800-1890). American cattle: their history, breeding, and management. **1868.** New York: Taintor Bros. 528 pp. §
   With 71 pp on diseases based on Clater.
011. **ALLEN, R.L. (Richard L.)** (1803-1869). Domestic animals: history and description of the horse, mule, cattle, sheep, swine, poultry, and farm dogs. **1847.** New York: O. Judd. 227 pp. §
   A farmers' handbook stressing management.
012.__Same. **1848.** New York: C.M. Saxton. 227 pp. §
013.__New American farm book. **1869.** New York: O. Judd. 526 pp.

Almanacs

014.__The American farmer's almanac. **1876.** Phila: Fisher & Bro. 34 pp. §
   Contains items of veterinary interest.
015.__The farmer's almanack. **1800.** Boston: John West. Unpaged. §
016.__Housekeeper's almanac. **1877.** Phila: Sower, Potts & Co. §
017.__Same. **1884.** Phila: Carey Bros. §
018.__Same. **1887.** Phila: Behm & Gerhart. §
019.__Knickerbocker's almanac. **1831.** New York: C. Brown. §
020.__The oracle of rural life: an almanack for sportsmen, farmers...for the year 1839. **1839.** London: A.H. Bailey. 96 pp. §
021.__Uncle Sam's almanac... **1844.** Phila: Hogan & Thompson. §
022.__Same. **1857.** Phila: Leary & Getz. 52 pp. §
023.__The Whig almanac. **1853.** New York: Greeley & McElrath. 65 pp. §
024.__Wright's pictorial family almanac. **1876.** New York: E. Ferratt. 24 pp. §
025.__Same. **1881.** §

---

026. **AMAR, Antonio**. Informe sobre la mejora y aumento de la cria de caballos dado al supremo consejo do la guerra... **1818.** Barcelona: Augustin Roca. 125 pp.
   Uses of horses in war.
027. **ANDERSEN, Sigurd** (ed). P.C. Abildgaard (1740-1801): a biography & bibliography for the faculty of veterinary science, the Royal Danish Veterinary and Agricultural University. **1985.** Copenhagen: Kandrup. 94 pp.
   The life and writings of the founder of the Danish veterinary school.

Animal Disease

028.__Farmer's cyclopedia. Abridged...from the publications of the United States Department of Agriculture. Volume 3 [of 7]: Diseases of cattle, sheep, goats, cats, dogs. **1915.** Garden City, NY: Doubleday, Page. 659 pp. §
   A generally sensible work for farmers.
029.__National Research Council...A historical survey of animal-disease morbidity and mortality reporting... **1966.** Washington: NAS-NRC. 40 pp. §
   Includes animal and human disease nomenclature.

030.__Rex book: the veterinary guide...treatments of the various diseases of horses, cattle, hogs, sheep and poultry. **1905** Omaha: The Rex Co. 160 pp. §

    A mediocre work promoting remedies.

031.__(Rinderpest) New York State Agricultural Society. First and second reports...on the statistics, pathology and treatment...of rinderpest. **1867**. Albany: Weed, Parsons. 144 pp.

    Based on European experience, with history.

032.__(Rinderpest) Report of...conference on diseases amongst cattle and other animals in South Africa... **1904**. Bloemfontein: Argus Printing. 66 pp.

    On rinderpest, TB, glanders, F&M disease, etc.

033.__(Tuberculosis) Report of...the outbreak of disease among the cattle at the state college farm... **1887**. Augusta, ME: Sprague & Son. 254 pp. §

    TB in the University of Maine dairy herd.

034.__Veterinary counter practice...including diseases and treatments... 9th ed. **1937**. London: Chemist and Druggist. 480 pp. §

    A mediocre work for the drug trade.

Animal Welfare; Vivisection

035.__**ALEXANDER, Lloyd.** Fifty years in the doghouse. **1964**. New York: Putnam. 256 pp.

    A narrative by New York SPCA agent No. 1.

036.__**ANGELL, George Thorndyke** (1823-1909). Autobiographical sketches and personal reflections. Boston: Am Humane Educ Soc. **1892?** 114 + 37 pp.

    An early SPCA leader; name associated with Angell Memorial (Animal) Hospital in Boston.

037.__Same: Second supplement. **1897**. 24 pp.

038.__**BAYLY, Maurice Beddow.** Clinical medical discoveries. **1961**. London: Natl Antivivisection Soc. 146 pp.

    Decries use of animals in medical research.

039.__The futility of experiments on animals. **1962**. (Same) 196 pp.

    Quotes selected to discredit such work.

040.__**BELL, Ernest** (1851-). Fair treatment for animals. **1927**. London: G. Bell & Sons. 298 pp.

    Several articles urging humane treatment.

041.__**BRAY, Caroline (Hennell)** (1814-1905). Our duty to animals. **1881**. London: S.W. Partridge. 160 pp.

    A children's book on humane treatment.

042.__**BROWN, Antony.** Who cares for animals. **1974**. London: Heinemann. 234 pp.

    A 150-year history of the RSPCA.

043.__**CIABURRI, G.** La vivisection. Trans from Italian by Robert Fath. **1928**. Geneva: Fed Swiss Soc against Vivisection. 288 pp.

    A condemnation of vivisection.

044.__CLARKE, Frances Elizabeth (ed). Poetry's plea for animals: an anthology... **1927**. Boston: Lothrop, Lee & Shepard. 426 pp.

A sentimental collection urging kindness.

045.__COBBE, Frances Power (1822-1904). The modern rack: papers on vivisection. **1893**. London: Swan, Sonnenschein. 272 pp. §

By founder of Natl Antivivisection Society.

046.__COLEMAN, Sydney R. Humane society leaders in America, with...early history of the humane movement in England. **1924**. Albany, NY: American Humane Assn. 270 pp.

Work of Henry Bergh, Geo T. Angell, et al.

047.__COLERIDGE, Stephen (1854-). Great testimony against scientific cruelty... **1918**. London; New York: John Lane Co. 66 pp.

Thoughts of famous persons on cruelty.

048.__COLLINS, John (1814?-1902). Voices of the dumb creation. A sequel to "Black Beauty." **1892**. Phila: Penna SPCA. 53 pp.

An allegorical convocation protesting cruelty.

049.__COLMORE, G(ertrude) (-1926). Priests of progress. **1908**. New York: B.W. Dodge. 384 pp.

A novel recounting horrors of vivisection.

050.__EVANS, Edward Payson (1831-1917). The criminal prosecution and capital punishment of animals. **1906**. London: W. Heinemann. 384 pp.

Medieval civil and clerical proceedings.

051.__FAIRHOLME, Edward George. A century of work for animals: the history of the RSPCA, 1824-1924. **1924**. New York: E.P. Dutton. 298 pp.

Founding of the RSPCA and its accomplishments.

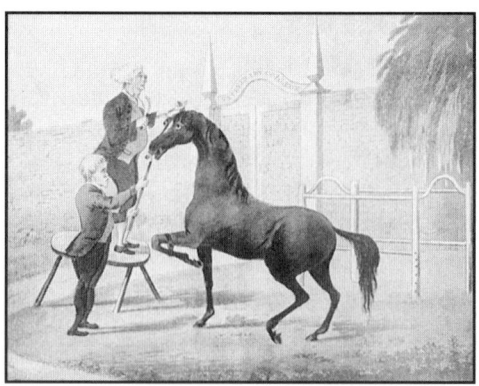

Fleming: The wanton mutilation of animals, 1898
(052)

052.__FLEMING, George (1833-1901). The wanton mutilation of animals. **1898**. London: George Bell & Sons. 24 pp; 10 plates.

Decries "fashionable" operations on animals.

053.__**FLETCHER, R.** A few notes on cruelty to animals: On the inadequacy of penal law... **1846**. London: Longman & Co. 105 pp.

    A plea for humane care; hospitalization.

054.__**FLOWER, Edward Fordham** (1805-1883). Bits and bearing-reins: with observations on horses and harness. **1885**. London: Cassell. 7th ed, 63 pp.

    Deplores use of the bearing-rein.

055.__**FOX, Michael W.** (1937-). Returning to Eden: animal rights and human responsibility. **1980**. New York: Viking Press. 281 pp.

    Implications of animal abuse for humanity.

056.__**FRENCH, R.D.** Antivivisection and medical science in Victorian society. **1975**. Princeton, NJ: Princeton Univ Press. 425 pp.

    Philosophy of the movement in Britain.

057.__**GALSWORTHY, John** (1867-1933). The slaughter of animals for food. **1913**. London: RSPCA Council of justice to animals. 24 pp.

    Urges stricter regulation of slaughter.

058.__**GOUGH, Edward W.** "Centaur," or, the "turn out": a practical treatise on the management of horses... **1878**. London: Hardwick & Bogue.

    Urges humane treatment; interesting plates.

059.__(**Humane movement**). Animal expression: a photographic footnote to Charles Darwin's "Expression of the emotions in man and animals." **1967**. New York: Animal Welfare Institute. 54 pp.

    Photos depicting joy, pain, terror, etc.

060.__ __Care and kindness for our animal friends. **1899**. American Humane Educ Soc. 30 pp.

    Introductory animal care for children.

061.__ __Corporation of London. Public Health Department report [on] humane slaughtering of animals. **1925**. London: Skipper & East. 16 pp.

062.__ __Dog welfare: a helpful book on dog ailments. **1900?** London: Natl Canine Defence League. 32 pp.

    A pamphlet for owners, ed by vet surgeon.

063.__ __Dundee SPCA annual report... **n.d.** Dundee, Scotland: John Leng & Co. 15 pp.

    Includes abridged reports of prosecutions.

064.__ __Great Britain. Anno Duodecimo...Anno primo...Anno quinto...[Three] act[s] for...prevention of cruelty to animals. **1849, 1837, 1835** London: G.E. Eyre & W. Spottiswood. 10, 2, 8 pp.

065.__ __A plea for the dumb creation: being selections from The British Workman, etc. **1868**. Phila: J.S. Claxton. 93 pp.

    Literary contributions and animal anecdotes.

066.__ __(same) **1876**. Penna SPCA. 96 pp.

067.__**HUME, C(harles) W(esley)** (1866-1981). The status of animals in Christian religion. **1956**. London: UFAW. 109 pp. §

    Early attitudes toward animals.

068.__**JACKSON, Thomas** (1812-1886). Our dumb companions, or, conversations of a father with his children... **1868**. London: S.W. Partridge. 134 pp.

A child's book stressing humane treatment.

069.__**KARKEEK, William Floyd** (1802-1858). An essay on the future existence of the brute creation. **1878**. London: W. Mitchell. 67 pp. §

Some early thoughts on the human-animal bond.

070.__**KEEN, William W(illiams)** (1837-). Animal experimentation and medical progress. **1914**. Boston; New York: Houghton Mifflin. 312 pp. §

Summarizes the benefits of vivisection.

071.__**LEAVITT, Emily Stewart.** Animals and their legal rights: a survey of American laws from 1641 to 1968...[with additions by USDA]. **1968**. New York: NY Anim Welfare Inst. 165 + 49 pp.

Evolution of laws to protect animals.

072.__**LEFFINGWELL, Albert** (1845-1916). An ethical problem: or, sidelights upon science experimentation on man and animals. **1914**. London: G. Bell & Sons; New York: C.P. Farrell. 369 pp.

Condemns animal research that is not "perfectly painless." Author signature.

073.__ __(same). **1916**. 374 pp.

074.__ __The vivisection controversy: essays and criticism. **1908**. London: The London and Provincial Anti-vivisection Society. 251 pp.

Disputes the claimed utility of vivisection.

075.__ __The vivisection question. **1907**. Chicago: Vivisection Reform Soc. 2nd ed. 267 pp.

A vehement objection to medical research.

076.__**LEWIS, C.S.** The problem of pain. **1974**. New York: Macmillan. paperback, 160 pp.

Includes section on animal pain.

077.__**MACAULAY, James** (1817-1902) et al. **1881**. Vivisection, scientifically and ethically considered in prize essays. London: M. Jaap. 317 pp.

Three essays on evils of vivisection.

078.__**MACNAGHTEN, Lettice.** Pistol v. poleaxe. A handbook on humane slaughter. **1932**. London: Chapman & Hall. 577 pp.

Slaughter methods and related legislation.

079.__**MUSHET, David** (1772-1847). The wrongs of the animal world... **1839**. London: Hatchard & Son. 324 pp.

Essays on animal cruelty and vivisection.

080.__**NIVEN, Charles D.** History of the humane movement. **1967**. New York: Transatlantic arts. 217 pp.

Development of thought about the movement.

081.__**OLDFIELD, Josiah** (1863-1963). The evils of butchery. **1895**. London: Wm Reeves. 77 + 21 pp.

A critique of killing methods.

082.__**PACE, Mildred Mastin.** Friend of animals: the story of Henry Bergh. **1942**. New York: C. Scribner's Sons. 125 pp.

Life of ASPCA founder, written for children.

083.__PAGET, Stephen (1855-1926). Experiments on animals. **1900**. London: T. Fisher Unwin. 274 pp.
    Refutes opponents of medical research.
084.__ __(same) **1903**. New York: G.P. Putnam's Sons. Revised ed. 380 pp.
085.__PATERSON, David; RYDER, Richard D. (ed). Animals' rights: a symposium. **1979**. London: Centaur Press. 243 pp.
    Social, historical and political perspective.
086.__PEABODY, Philip Glendower (1857-). Personal experiences of two American anti-vivisectionists...with an appendix by Col. Robert G. Ingersoll. **1895**. Boston: New England Anti-vivisection Society. 96 pp.
    Perceived horrors, mainly in Europe.
087.__(Periodicals). The animal world. Vol 3, No 25. **1908**. London: H.E. Morgan. 290 pp.
    Monthly publication of the RSPCA.
088.__ __National humane review. Vol 50, No 1. 50th anniversary issue. **1962**. §
    Articles on origins of humane movement.
089.__PHILANTHROPOS (pseud). Physiological cruelty, or...an inquiry into the vivisection question. **1883**. New York: John Wiley. 156 pp.
    Comes down in favor of animal experiments.
090.__PLIMSOLL, Samuel (1824-1898). Cattle ships...Mr. Plimsoll's second appeal for our seamen... **1890**. London: K. Paul, Trench. 150 pp.
    Overloading and ship loss; Plimsoll line.
091.__REGAN, Tom. The case for animal rights. **1983**. Berkeley: Univ Calif Press. 425 pp.
    A philosophic inquiry; human obligations.
092.__ROWLEY, Francis Harold (1854-). The humane idea: a brief history of man's attitude toward the other animals. **1912**. Boston: American Humane Educ Soc. 72 pp.
    Early concepts and related legislation.
093.__RYDER, Richard D(udley). Victims of science: the use of animals in research. **1975**. London: Davis-Poynter. 279 pp.
    Claims most animal experimentation is trivial.
094.__SALT, Henry Stephens (1851-1939). Animals' rights: considered in relation to social progress. **1892**. London; New York: G. Bell. 162 pp.
    A plea for humane treatment, wild and tame.
095.__ __(same) **1894**. New York. 176 pp.
    Includes essay by Albert Leffingwell.
096.__ __(same)...with preface by Peter Singer. **1980**. Clarks Summit, PA: Society for Animal Rights. 232 pp.
    Reprint, with extensive bibliography.
097.__SINGER, Peter. Animal liberation: a new ethics for our treatment of animals. **1973**. New York: Random House. 301 pp.
    Tyranny of human over nonhuman animals.
098.__SWALLOW, William Alan. Quality of mercy: history of the humane movement in the United States. **1963**. Boston: Mary Mitchell Humane Fund. 187 pp.

The work of numerous societies in the US.

099.__TRIST, Sidney (ed). The under dog: a series...on the wrongs suffered by animals... **1913**. London: "Animals' Guardian" Office. 203 pp.

Papers on docking, slaughter, bearing rein.

100.__TURNER, E(rnest) S(ackville) (1909-). All heaven in a rage. **1965**. New York: St Martin's Press. 324 pp.

Development of humane movement in Britain.

101.__TURNER, James (1946-). Reckoning with the beast: animals, pain, and humanity in the Victorian mind. **1980**. Baltimore: Johns Hopkins Univ. 190 pp.

Sociology of the humane movement.

102.__(Vivisection). Great Britain...return showing the number of experiments on living animals. **1915, 1920**. London: HMSO. 27, 34 pp.

Lists of experimenters and animal types.

103.__ __Royal commission on vivisection, fifth report...appendix. **1908**. London: HMSO. 4 + 157 pp.

Official forms and index of evidence given.

104.__ __(same). Final report. **1912**. 139 pp.

Justification for animal experimentation.

105.__ __[Minor publications] **1895-1946**.

Pro and con, 55 small items.

106.__ __US Congress. [Senate hearing on bill for prevention of cruelty to animals.] **1900**. Washington: GPO. 223 pp. §

Includes statements by prominent persons.

107.__ __World League against vivisection. Fourth international congress. **1910**. London: J. Tamblyn. 357 pp.

Short papers by congress participants.

108.__WARBASSE, James Peter (1866-1957). The conquest of pain through animal experimentation. **1910**. New York; London: D. Appleton. 175 pp. §

The role of animals in medical progress.

109.__WESTACOTT, Evalyn (1888-). A century of vivisection and anti-vivisection...their effect upon science, medicine and human life... **1949**. Ashingdon, Essex: C.W. Daniel. 675 pp. §

A largely one-sided "expose" of research.

---

110. ANTRIM, A.A. The horseman's friend. **1878**. Logan, IA: [s.n.] 27 pp.

Tidbits of information, eg, colic, big head.

APPERLY, Charles—see Nimrod

111. ARBURUA, Joseph M. Narrative of the veterinary profession in California. **1966**. San Francisco: [s.n.]. 366 pp.§

Organizations, education, DVM biographies.

112. (ARISTOTLE). Aristotle's history of animals. **1907**. London: G. Bell & Sons. 326 pp. §

Includes his books on parts of animals, internal organs, reproduction and diseases.

113. **ARMATAGE, George.** Every man his own horse doctor...[with] Blaine's veterinary art... **1877?** New York: O. Judd. 830 pp. §
   Early mention of some conditions, eg, roaring.
114.___Memoranda for emergencies, or, the veterinarian's pocket remembrancer. **1870.** London: J. Churchill & Sons. 262 pp. §
   Diagnosis and treatment of acute conditions.
115.___The sheep: its varieties and management in health and disease. **1882.** London: F. Warne. 211 pp. §
   A comprehensive handbook for shepherds.
116.___The thermometer as an aid to diagnosis in veterinary medicine. **1894.** London: F. Warne. 71 pp.
   A pioneering work on the subject.
117. **ARMSTEAD, Hugh W.** The artistic anatomy of the horse. **1900.** London: Bailliere, Tindall. 48 pp.
   Detailed but superficial and inelegant.
118. **ASH, Edward Cecil** (1888-). Dogs: their history and development. **1900?** Boston: Houghton Mifflin. 2 vol, 384, 394 pp. §
   Early writings, with elegant plates of breeds.
   ASHMONT—see Perry, Joseph.
119. **AVERY, James** (1809-). Old Jim Avery's own farrier and recipe book...for the prevention and cure of disease in horses. **1859.** Albany, NY: Munsell & Rowland. 340 pp. §
   Some good observations, except on disease.
120. **AXE, J. Wortley** (ed). The horse, its treatment in health and disease, with a complete guide to breeding, training, and management. **1906.** London: Gresham Publishing Co. 9 vol, 1605 pp. §
   An encyclopedic work; many illustrations.
121. **BABCOCK, Robert H(all)** (1851-). Diseases of the heart and arterial system... **1903.** New York; London: D. Appleton. 853 pp. §
   A text for students and physicians.
122. **BACON, Francis** (1561-1626). Sylva sylvarum. **1658.** London: W. Rawley. 125 pp. §
   A late edition of Bacon's natural history. [Bound with] New Atlantis. **1658.** 36 pp, [and] The history of life and death. **1658.** 62 pp. Latter includes ages to which animals live.
   BADCOCK, J.—see Hinds, John
123. **BAKER, Austin Hart** (1852-). Live stock: a cyclopedia for the farmer and stock owner...being also a complete stock doctor. **1912.** Minneapolis: H.L. Baldwin. 1406 pp.
   Well-written, many illustrations; by dean of Chicago Veterinary College.
124.___(same). **1918.** c1916. Detroit: F.B. Dickerson. 1404 pp. §
125.___Theory and practice of veterinary medicine... **1909.** 2nd ed. Chicago: A. Eger. 265 pp. §
   Based on author's lecture notes.
126. **BAKER, E.T.** Sheep diseases. **1916.** Chicago: Amer J Vet Med. 237 pp. §
   Includes color plates of poisonous plants.

127.__(same) Chicago: Alex Eger. 299 pp. §
   Revised edition without color plates.
128. **BALLMER, D.** Neue Recepte und bewahrte Curen fur Menschen und Vieh. **1827**. Schellsburg, PA: [s.n.]. 40 pp. §
   Cures for man and cattle; 30 pp missing.
129. **BALLOU, William Rice** (1864-1893). A compend of equine anatomy and physiology. **1890**. Phila: P. Blakiston. 205 pp. §
   A quiz compendium and dissection guide.
130. **(BANG)** Bernhard Lauritz Frederik (1848-1932). Lagen og veterinaeren, der forte Dansk veterinaervidenskab... **1984**. Kobenhavn: Carl Fr. Mortensens Forlag. 101 pp. §
   The Danish veterinarian noted for his work on bovine abortion (Bang's disease) and TB. With Hist Med Vet 5:3 (Letters to Bang).
131. **BANHAM George Amos.** Table of veterinary posology and therapeutics...for the use of students and practitioners. **1901**. New York: W.R. Jenkins. 192 pp.
   Tables of medications and diseases; remedies.
132.__(same) **1901**. London: Bailliere, Tindall.
133. **BARDSLEY, Samuel Argent** (1764-1851). Medical reports of cases and experiments, with...an enquiry into the origin of canine madness... **1807**. London: R. Bickerstaff. 336 pp. §
   Includes anecdotes of "spontaneous" rabies.
134. **BARKER, C(lifford) A(lbert) V(ictor)** (1919-). One voice: a history of the Canadian Veterinary Medical Association. **1989**. Ottawa: CVMA. 260 pp. §
   Includes veterinary education; biographies.
135. **BARKLEY, K.** The ambulance. **1978**. Hicksville, NY: Exposition Press. 207 pp. §
   Includes animal ambulances. Inscribed by author to J.F. Smithcors.
136. **BARNUM, H.L.** The American farrier: containing a minute account of...every part of the horse. **1832**. Phila: U. Hunt; Cincinnati: H.L. Barnum. 286 pp.
   A generally sensible work for owners.
137.__(same) **1845**. c1832. Phila: U. Hunt. §
138. **BARTLET, J(ohn)** (1716?-1772). The gentleman's farriery, or, a practical treatise on the diseases of horses. **1754**. 2nd ed. London: J. Nourse. 370 pp.
   By a surgeon with little knowledge of horses.
139.__(same) **1770**. 7th ed. §
140.__(same) **1773**. 8th ed. §
141.__(same) **1782**. 10th ed. C. Nourse. §
142.__(same) **1788**. 12th ed. §
143.__Pharmacopoeia Bartleiana, or, Bartlet's gentleman farrier's repository... **1773**. Eton: T. Pote. 400 pp.
   Essentially a reprint of item 144.
144.__Pharmacopoeia hippiatrica, or, the gentleman farrier's repository... **1764**. Eton: J. Pote. 382 pp. §
   Based on item 138; not a pharmacopoeia.

145. **BARTON, William P(aul) C(rillon)** (1786-1856). Vegetable materia medica of the United States... **1817, 1818.** Phila: M. Carey. 2 vol, 273, 243 pp.

A descriptive work, with fine color plates.

146. **BASKIN, Leonard** (1922-). Ars anatomica: a medical fantasia. **1972.** New York: Medicina Rara. §

Thirteen contemporary drawings 16 x 22."

147. **BAUM, H(ermann)** (1864-1932). Das Lymphgefasssystem des Rindes. **1912.** Berlin: A. Hirschwald. 170 pp.

The bovine lymphatic system; 32 color plates.

148. **BAYER, Joseph.** Lehrbuch der Veterinarchirurgie. **1887.** Wien: W. Eraumuller. 536 pp.

A general veterinary surgery textbook.

149. **BEASLEY, Henry.** The druggist's general receipt book...veterinary formulary...materia medica...proprietary medicines, [etc]... **1857.** Phila: Lindsay & Blakiston. 3rd Amer ed. 495 pp.

Has 150 pp on veterinary drugs; medications.

150. **BEAUMONT, T(homas).** The complete cow doctor: being a treatise on the disorders incident to horned cattle...by T. Beamont [sic]. **1814.** Leeds: G. Wilson. 108 pp.

Poor, except for appendix on parturition.

151. __The complete new cow doctor...to which is added a concise treatise on farriery. **1835.** Manchester: S. Johnson. 140 pp.

Pp 97-140 are devoted to farriery.

152. **BECKFORD, Peter** (1740-1811). Thoughts on hunting: in a series of familiar letters to a friend. **1810.** London: J. Cundee. 314 pp. §

Kennel diseases, by an observant layman.

153. __(same) **1951.** London: Methuen. 220 pp. §

154. **BELL, Charles, Sir** (1774-1842). Manuscript of drawings of the arteries. **1971?** New York: Editions Medicina Rara, facsimile 1797 ed.

With many colored plates and commentary.

155. **BENION, AD.** Traite de l'elevage et des maladies du porc. **1872.** Paris: P. Asselin. 539 pp.§

Written to lessen indifference of DVMs. Has extensive history of cysticercosis.

156. **BENNION, Elisabeth.** Antique medical instruments. **1979.** London: Sotheby Parke Bernet; Berkeley, CA: Univ Calif Press. 355 pp.

Includes veterinary items, middle ages to 1870; copiously illustrated.

157. **BENTWRIGHT, Jeremiah.** The American horse tamer...stable economy: and remedies for all diseases to which horses are liable... **1858.** New York: A.O. Moore. 86 pp. §

Mentions glanders, distemper, lampas, etc.

158. **BERENGER, Richard.** A new system of horsemanship. **1754.** London: Paul Vaillant. 147 pp. §

Trans of Bourgelat's "The new Newcastle," in turn trans (from English) of monumental work of Wm Cavendish, Duke of Newcastle (1667).

159. **BERJEAU, Ph. Charles.** The horses of antiquity, middle ages, and the renaissance. **1864.** London: Dulau & Co. §
   Sixty drawings with text, to 16th century.
160. **BERNERS, Juliana** (1388-). The boke of Saint Albans...containing treatises on hawking, hunting, and cote armour... **1881.** London: E. Stock, facsimile 1486 ed; introduction by Wm Blades. 32 pp + 90 leaves facsimiles. §
   First printed English work with vet import.
161. **BEYER, B.** Viehseuchen-Gesetze...uber die Abwehr und Unterdrucking von Viehseuchen. **1886.** Berlin: P. Parey. 360 pp.
   State regulation of livestock in Germany.
162. **BIERER, Bert W.** American veterinary history. **1980.** Madison, WI: C. Olson. 220 pp. §
   From 18th to 20th century; 729 references; author signature; letter to J.F. Smithcors.
163. __History of animal plagues of North America... **1974** c1939. Washington: USDA. 97 pp. §
   A chronology of disease outbreaks 1700-1939.
164. __A short history of veterinary medicine in America. **1955.** East Lansing: Michigan State Univ Press. 118 pp. §
   Animal plagues and the rise of vet medicine.
165. **BIGGLE, Jacob.** Biggle swine book: much old and more new knowledge... **1899.** Phila: Wilmer Atkinson Co. 144 pp. §
   Swine husbandry and diseases.
166. **BILLINGS, Frank Seaver** (1845-1912). The relation of animal diseases to the public health, and their prevention. **1884.** New York: D. Appleton. 446 pp.
   A pioneering work; sections on veterinary history and schools of Europe.
167. **BINDLEY, Charles** (1796-1859) (pseud for Harry Hieover). The pocket and the stud, or, practical hints on the management of the stable. **1851.** London: Longman, Brown... 218 pp. §
   Largely sensible; with advice to purchasers.
168. **BINNIE, John Fairbairn** (1863-). Manual of operative surgery. **1911.** Phila: P. Blakiston's Sons. 5th ed, 1153 pp.
   A comprehensive basic human surgery text.
169. **BIRCH, Raymond H.** Hog cholera: its nature and control. **1922.** New York: Macmillan. 311 pp.
   Diagnosis and treatment of hog cholera.
170. **BLACKLOCK, Ambrose** (1816-1873). A treatise on sheep...their improvement...management...treatment of their diseases... **1841.** London: R. Tyas. 236 pp.
   Scientific and practical, except on rot.
171. **BLAGRAVE, Joseph** (1610-1682). The epitome of the art of husbandry...directions for the improvement of it... **1675.** London: R. Billingsley. 236 + 136 pp.
   Sections on animal disease and horsemanship.

Delabere Pritchett Blaine

172.__Canine pathology, or...the diseases of dogs: with their causes, symptoms and mode of cure. **1817.** London: T. Boosey 326 pp. §
  Established Blaine as "father" of discipline.

173.__(same) **1824.** London: Boosey & Sons. 326 pp. §
  With "copious detail of the rabid malady."

174.__(same) **1832.** London: T. & T. Boosey. 316 pp. §

175.__Blaine's canine pathology: being a description of the diseases of dogs... **1851.** London: Longman, Brown... 5th ed, rev by Thomas Walton Mayer. 236 pp.
  An updated version of Blaine's work.

176.__A domestic treatise on the diseases of horses and dogs. **1803.** London: T. Boosey. 212 pp.§
  A do-it-yourself work touting his remedies; a gift from the author to Colonel Fall.

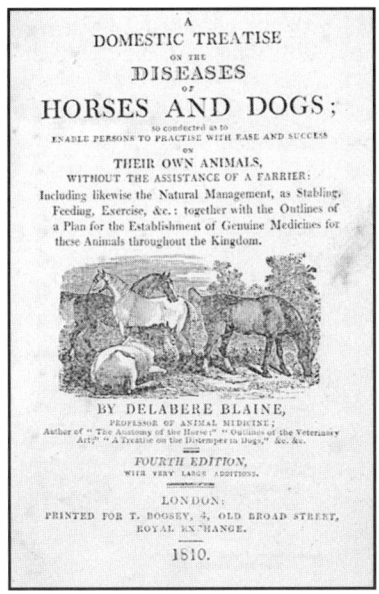

Blaine: 1810 (177)

177.__(same) **1810.** 4th ed, 249 pp.

178.__An encyclopaedia of rural sports... **1852.** London: Longman, Brown... rev ed by Harry Hieover. 1246 pp. §
  A scholarly work, with many references.

179.__The outlines of the veterinary art, or, the principles of medicine as applied to...the horse, the ox, the sheep,and the dog, and to...their various diseases. **1802**. London: Longman & Rees. 2 vol, 560, 783 pp. §

Reflects inexperience of a human surgeon; includes vet history, views of education.

180.__(same) **1816**. London: T. Boosey. 2nd ed, 314 + 128 pp. §

Lacks part 3 on diseases; section on animal physiology added (author?).

181.__The outlines of the veterinary art, or, a treatise on the anatomy, physiology, and curative treatment of the horse...neat cattle and sheep. **1832**. London: Longman. 4th ed. 668 pp. §

Greatly improved over earlier editions.

182.__(same) **1841**. London: Longman, Orme. 5th ed, 643 pp. §

183.__(same) **1865**. London: Longmans, Green... 7th ed, rev and enl by Charles Steel. 814 pp. §

---

184. **BLAZE, Elsear Jean Louis Joseph** (1786-1848). Le chasseur au chien d'arret...l'education des chiens, leur maladies... **1836**. Paris: Moutardier. 424 pp. §

The education and maladies of hunting dogs.

185. **BONSI, Francesco** (1722-1803). Il dilettante di cavalli istruito... **1757**. Venezia: G. Occhi. 68 pp.

Anatomy, diseases and treatment of horses.

186.__Istruzione veterinaria...sulla presente epidemia contagiosa de' buoi... **1786**. Rimino: Stamperia Albertiniana. 71 pp.

An early work on cattle plague.

187. **BOURGELAT, Claude** (1710-1799). Elemens de l'art veterinaire: traite de la conformation exterieure du cheval. **1803**. Paris: Huzard. 5th ed, 580 pp.

A monumental work on the horse.

188.__Matiere medicale raisonnee du precis des medicamens consideree dans leur effets... **1765**. Lyon: J.M. Bruyset. 239 pp. §

By the head of the first French school (1761).

189. **BOURGUIGNON, Honore.** On the cattle plague...history, origin, description, and treatment. **1869**. Phila: J.B. Lippincott. 379 pp. §

A major work on rinderpest, incl prevention.

190. **BOWKER, G.H.** How to keep a house dog... **n.d.** London: Natl Canine Defence League. 32 pp.

A pamphlet for owners.

Henry Bracken (1697-1764)

191. (__) Every man his own farrier: containing ten minutes advice how to buy a horse...remedies for...all diseases to which he is liable. **1843**, Phila: J.B. Perry; New York: Nafis & Cornish. 98 pp.

A plagiarism of Bracken, Burden and Taplin.

192.__Farriery improv'd...wherein is fully explain'd the nature, structure, and mechanism of a horse: the diseases and accidents he is liable to... **1737**. London: J. Clarke. 616 pp. §

By a physician with little equine experience.

193.__(same) **1738**. 363 pp.
194.__(same) **1739**. 363 pp.
195.__(same) **1756**. London: J. Shuckburgh. 363 pp.

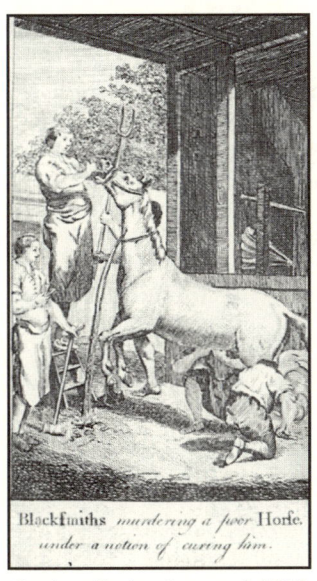

Bracken: Farriery improved, 1796
(196)

196.__(same) **1796**. Phila: M. Carey. 144 pp. §

Abridged from the 1737 ed, with 10 folding plates and sections on other animals added.

197.__Taplin improved...[rest of title as for item 192]. **1815**. Troy, NY: F. Adancourt... 204 pp. §

Based on Taplin 1811 ed but attributed to Bracken, with American data added.

198.__The traveler's pocket farrier, or, a treatise upon the distempers and common incidents happening to horses upon a journey... **1744**. London: B. Dod. 150 pp. §

Based on Burdon: the Gentleman's Pocket Farrier (qv) and published under that title by Bracken (London 1735).

199.__(same) **1750**. London: Dod & Johnston. 150 pp.
200.__(same) **1755**. 150 pp.

201. **BRADLEY, O(rlando) Charnock** (1871-1937). History of the Edinburgh Veterinary College. **1923**. Edinburgh: Oliver & Boyd. 101 pp. §
Centennial volume of the Edinburgh school.

202. __Topographic anatomy of the dog. **1943**. New York: Macmillan. 4th ed, 316 pp.
Useful as dissection guide; E.A. Ehmer's copy.

203. **BRADLEY, Richard** (1688-1732). The gentleman and farmer's guide for the increase and improvement of cattle...horses... **1729**. London: W. Mears. 352 pp. §
Good on sheep rot; reference to hog cholera?

204. **BRETON, F.; LARIEUX, E.** Les maladies du cheval: (elements de clinique veterinaire). **1923**. Paris: Vigot Freres. 498 pp. §
Medical and surgical conditions of horses; includes iv and sc oxygen therapy.

205. **BROWN, Thomas M.P.S.** A manual of modern farriery: embracing the cure of diseases incidental to horses, cattle...instructions in racing [etc]... **1846?** London: G. Virtue. 920 pp. §
Intended to combat quackery by owners.

206. **BROWN, Thomas.** An inquiry into the antivariolous power of vaccination... **1809**. Edinburgh: G. Ramsay. 327 pp.
Discovery and early experiences.

207. **BROWN, W.W.; BROWN, D.** A hundred years of veterinary medicine in Illinois 1882-1982. **1982**. Aurora, IL: Illinois VMA. 162 pp. §
State organizations, education and practice; inscribed by authors to J.F. Smithcors.

208. **BROWNE, John** (1642-1700?). Myographia nova, or, a description of all the muscles in the humane body... **1971?** New York: Editions Medicina Rara. Facsimile 1697 ed. 109 pp, 38 plates. §
A detailed dissection of the muscles

209. **BROWNE, Peter A(rrell)** (1782-1860). An essay on the veterinary art...the veterinary colleges in France and England...and utility of instituting similar schools in the United States. **1837**. Phila: J. Thompson. 22 pp.
A plea for veterinary schools in America.

210. **BRUGNONE, Carlo Giovanni** (1741-1818). Trattato delle razze de' cavalli. **1781**. Torino: Fratelli Reycends. 564 pp.
Management and diseases of the horse.

211. **BRUMDER, George.** Der Hausthier-Arzt, fur den amerikanischen Farmer und Viehzuchter... **1886**. Milwaukee: G. Brumder. 375 pp.
Animal disease, cattle breeding, obstetrics.

212. **BRUMLEY, Oscar Victor.** Book of veterinary posology and prescriptions. **1913**. Columbus, OH: R.G. Adams. 190 pp.
A handbook of medications and doses.

213.__(same) **1924**. rev ed, 213 pp.

214.__A text-book of the diseases of the small domestic animals. **1931**. Phila: Lea & Febiger. 2nd ed, 611 pp. §
A long-standard text; 2nd copy E.A. Ehmer's.

215. **BRUNSCHWIG, Hieronymus** (ca 1450-1512). Dis ist das Buch der Cirurgia...Wund Artzny. **1971?** New York: Medicina Rara. Facsimile 1500? ed. §
   Facsimile of early work on wound treatment.
216. **BRUSH. H.D.** A new system of horse training or horse education. **1900?** Toronto: Carswell. 224 pp. §
   System of horsemanship; lameness treatment.
217. **BRYCE, James.** Practical observations on the inoculation of cowpox...test of perfect vaccination... **1809.** Edinburgh: W. Creech. 2nd ed, 132 pp.
   History of cowpox; early vaccination attempts.
218. **BUCHAN, William** (1729-1805). Every man his own doctor... **1816.** New Haven, CT: N. Whiting. 464 + 144 pp. §
   From Buchan's Domestic Medicine (London 1769) with retrograde section on farriery added.
219. **BUCHANAN, Robert E.; MURRAY, Charles.** Veterinary bacteriology. A treatise on the bacteria, yeasts, molds, and protozoa pathogenic for domestic animals. **1922.** Phila: W.B. Saunders. 3rd ed, 606 pp. §
220. **BULLOCK, Fred** (1878-). Handbook for veterinary surgeons. **1936.** London: Bailliere Tindall & Cox. 302 pp.
   British law relating to veterinary practice.
221. **BURDON, William** (-1732?). The gentleman's pocket farrier: shewing how to use your horse on a journey and what remedies are proper for common misfortunes that may befal him on the road. **1730.** London: The author. 101 pp. §
   By an early advocate of humane treatment.
222. __The gentleman's pocket farrier...with remarks by Dr. Henry Bracken... **1735.** London: J. Clarke. 3rd ed, 78 pp.
223. __(same). **1748.** London: W. Johnston. 4th ed, 76 pp. §
224. __The gentleman's pocket farrier: showing how to use a horse on a journey and what remedies are proper for common accidents that may befal him on the road. **1823.** Phila: T. Desilver. 50 pp.
   An Americanized abridgement of Burdon's work.
225. **BURKE, B.W.** A compendium of the anatomy, physiology, and pathology of the horse. **1806.** Phila: J. Humphreys. 292 pp. §
   Mediocre, but advocates humane treatment.
226. **BURKETT, Charles William** (1873-). The farmer's veterinarian: a practical treatise on the diseases of farm stock... **1909.** New York: O. Judd. 275 pp. §
   Generally sensible advice for owners.
227. __(same): **1914.** 275 pp. §
228. **BURNETT, Samuel Howard** (1869-). The clinical pathology of the blood of domesticated animals. **1908.** Ithaca, NY: Taylor & Carpenter. 156 pp. §
   Details of blood in health and disease.
229. **BURNHAM, George P.** The history of the hen fever. A humorous record. **1855.** Boston: James French. 326 pp. §
   A satire on mania over exotic chickens.
230. **CADIOT, Pierre Juste** (1858-). Exercises in equine surgery. Trans by A.W. Bitting; ed by A. Liautard. **1897.** New York: W.R. Jenkins. 122 pp. §
   A early text for American students.

231.__Precis de chirurgie veterinaire. **1926**. Paris: Vigot Freres. 5th ed, 647 pp. §
  Surgery of all species; many illustrations.
232.__Roaring in horses, its pathology and treatment. Trans by T.J.W. Dollar. **1892**. New York: W.R. Jenkins. 78 pp. §
  Details treatment by arytenoidectomy.
233.__; ALMY, J. Traite de therapeutique chirurgicale des animaux domestiques. **1923**. Paris: Vigot Freres. 3rd ed, 1128 pp. §
  General and regional surgery; references.
234.__; BRETON, F. Medecine et chirurgie canines. **1924**. Paris: Asselin et Houzeau. 4th ed, 420 pp. §
  Specific medications; lacks surgical detail.
235. **CAIUS, John** (1510-1573). Of English dogges. **1880**. Reprint of 1576 ed. 44 pp.
  Fleming trans of De canibus Britannicus (1570) on types of English dogs.
236. **CAMPBELL, D(elwin) M(orton)** (1880-) (ed). Colics and their treatment. **1914**. Chicago: Am J Vet Med. 137 pp. §
237.__(same) **1915**. 2nd ed, 141 pp.
  E.A. Ehmer signature.
238.__Spring-time surgery. **1912**. Chicago: Am J Vet Med. 143 pp. §
239.__(same) **1912**. 2nd ed, 163 pp. §
240.__(same) **1913**. 3rd ed. 163 pp. §
241.__ (same) **1916**. 5th ed. 163 pp.
  E.A. Ehmer signature.
242.__Essentials of parasitology, including a brief discourse on zoology. **1907**. Hiawatha, KS: E. Herbert. 87 pp. §
  Taxonomy of parasites of domestic animals.
243. **CAMPBELL, James B.** The horse: diseases of his feet, care, treatment & cure of same. **1891**. Chicago: The author. 48 pp.
  A promotion of the author's foot remedies.
244. **CANFIELD, Henry Judson** (1789-1856). The breeds, management, structure and diseases of the sheep. **1848**. Salem, OH: A. Hinchman. 395 pp.
  Husbandry, with mediocre section on disease.
245. **CARPENTER, William Benjamin** (1813-1885). Animal physiology: a comprehensive sketch of the principal forms of animal structure. **1884**. London: W.S. Orr. 579 pp.
  A general text emphasizing lower forms.
246. **CARPENTIER, G.** Parasites et maladies parasitaires des equides domestiques. **1939**. Paris: Vigot Freres. 524 pp. §
  Classification, diagnosis, treatment and prevention; L.A. Merillat signature.
247. **CARRIER, E(lse) H(aydon)** (1879-). The pastoral heritage of Britain: a geographical study. **1936**. London: Christophers. 293 pp. §
  Social ecology of sheep and dairy farming.

248. **CARSON, James Crawford** (1815?-1886). The form of the horse, as it lies open to the inspection of the ordinary observer. **1862.** London: Simkin, Marshall and Co. 158 pp. §
   Some relationships of defects to disease.
249. **CARTER, William Giles Harding** (1851-). The horses of the world... **1923.** Washington: National Geographic Soc. 118 pp. §
   Breed histories, with many illustrations.
250.__Horses, saddles and bridles. **1906.** Baltimore: Lord Baltimore Press. 405 pp.
   Stable management of cavalry horses.
251. **CARVER, James.** Carver's repository, forge and horse infirmary... **1816?** New York: [s.n.]. 32 pp. §
   A proposal for instructing shoeing smiths, etc.
252.__The farrier's magazine, or, archives of veterinary science... **1818.** Phila: The author. 122 pp. §
   First US veterinary "journal;" 2 issues, but depicts contemporary conditions.
253. **CARVER, William.** Practical horse farriery...shewing the best method to preserve the horse in health; and...cure...of diseases... **1820.** Phila: M'Carty & Davis. 251 pp. §
   Sound writing by an experienced practitioner.
254. **CASSERI, Giulio Cesare** (1552-1616). Tabulae anatomicae LXXIIX... **1971?** New York: Editions Medicina Rara. Facsimile 16thC ed. §
   Facsimile of 16thC work on human anatomy.

Catalogs

255.__Alexander Eger: tenth annual catalogue of veterinary books and supplies. **1900?** Chicago: A. Eger. 64 pp.
   Complete book listing with specimen pages.
256.__Arnold & Sons: catalogue of veterinary instruments... **1893.** London: Arnold. 216 pp.
   Well illustrated, with prices.
257.__(same) **1902?** 303 pp.
258.__Haussmann & Dunn: catalogue...veterinary instruments and supplies... **1902?** Chicago: [s.n.]. 8th ed, 783 pp. §
   Includes textbooks, grinding services, etc.
259.__(same) **1916?** 15th ed, 767 pp.
260.__Haver-Glover Laboratories: catalog. **1928.** Kansas City: Burd & Fletcher. 3rd ed, 340 pp.
   Instruments and drugs, with prices.
261.__(same) **1930.** 4th ed, 400 pp.
262.__J.F. De Vine Laboratories: catalogue of pharmaceutical specialties and biological products. **1930?** Goshen, NY: J.F. De Vine Labs. 47 pp.

263.__J.H. Tuttle...price list of books, prints & horse goods... **1885**? New York: J.H. Tuttle. 53 pp.
    Includes surgical instruments.
264.__Jensen-Salsbery Laboratories: Jen-Sal biological catalog. **1927**. Kansas City: Jen-Sal Labs. 3rd ed, 96 pp.
265.__ __Jen-Sal instrument catalog. **1927**. Kansas City: Jen-Sal Labs. 3rd ed, 96 pp.
266.__ __Jen-Sal pharmaceutical catalog. **1928**. Kansas City: Jen-Sal Labs. 3rd ed, 104 pp. §
267.__ __The Jensalogue. **1929**. Kansas City: Jen-Sal Labs. 5th ed, 342 pp. §
268.__Max Wocher & Son: illustrated catalogue of veterinary instruments, books, drugs... **1910**? Cincinnati: Max Wocher. 14th ed, 272 pp.
269.__Neverslip Horseshoe Co: catalog. **1890**? Boston: [s.n.]. 48 pp. §
270.__Parke, Davis & Co: catalogue of...veterinary products... **1917**. Detroit: Parke, Davis. 134 pp.
271.__ __Veterinary materia medica. **1921**. London: Parke, Davis. 202 pp. §
272.__Pitman-Moore Co: descriptive catalogue...of...pharmaceutical and biological products... **1922**. Indianapolis: Pitman-Moore. 201 pp. §
273.__Royal College of Veterinary Surgeons: a catalogue of the books, pamphlets and periodicals up to 1850 in the library. **1965**. Supplement to Veterinary Record, May 1, 48 pp. §
274.__ __Catalog of the historical collection: books published before 1850. **1953**. Norwich: Jarrold & Sons. 36 pp. §
    With 6 p supplement (typescript) 1959.
275.__Sharp and Smith: catalog of veterinary surgical instruments. **1890**? Chicago: Sharp & Smith. 171 pp.
    Copiously illustrated.

---

276. (**CATO, Marcus Porcius**) (234-149 BC). Cato, the censor, on farming. Trans by Ernest Brehaut. **1933**. New York: Columbia Univ Press. 45 + 156 pp. §
    Roman husbandry, with sections on disease.
277. (**Cattle disease**). Bericht der...Vieh-seuche...recepten fuer dieselbe... **1682**. Braunschweig: Christoff-Friedrich Zilligern. 15 pp.
    An early work on cattle disease.
278.__The home cow doctor. **1927**. Lyndonville, VT: [s.n.]. 32 pp. §
    A pamphlet promoting dairy remedies.
279. (**Cattle industry**) Historical and biographical record of the cattle industry. **1959**. New York: Antiquarian Press. 2 vol, 293; 180 pp.
    Includes chapter on Texas fever.
    CAVEAT EMPTOR—see Stephen, George
280. **CHAMBERLAND, Ch.** (1851-). Le charbon et la vaccination charbonneuse d'apres les travaux recents de M. Pasteur. **1863**. Paris: B. Tignol. 316 pp.
    Pasteur's work on anthrax, by an associate.
281. **CHARLES IX, King of France** (1550-1574). La chasse royale. **1857**. Paris: Mm Bouchard-Huzard. 136 pp.
    Hunting during the 16th century.

282. **CHASE, A(lvin) W(ood)** (1817-1885). Dr Chase's recipes, or, information for everyone... **1866**. Ann Arbor, MI: The author. 33rd ed, 384 pp. §
   Includes "sure remedies" for horses.
283. **CHAUVEAU, Auguste** (1827-1917). The comparative anatomy of the domesticated animals. Trans and ed by George Fleming. **1884?** New York: W.R. Jenkins. 2nd ed, 957 pp. §
284.__(same) **1905**. New York: D. Appleton. 1084 pp.
285.__(same) **1906**.
286. **CHAWNER, Robert.** Diseases of the horse, and how to treat them... **1874**. Phila: Porter and Coates. 180 pp.
   An early work with rudiments of pathology.
287. **CHEEK, Henry.** Cheek's farriery...diseases of the horse, and their remedies. **1845**. St Louis: Reveille Press. 80 pp.
   An undistinguished work from various sources.
288. **CHENEVIX-TRENCH, Charles Pocklington** (1914-). A history of horsemanship. **1970**. Garden City, NY: Doubleday. 320 pp. §
   Ancient times to 20thC; many illustrations.
289. **CHENU, J.C.; DES MURS, O.** La fauconnerie ancienne et moderne. **1862**. Paris: Librarie Hachette. 176 pp. §
   Breeds and management of falcons.
290. **CHIODI, Valentino.** Storia della veterinaria. **1957**. Milano: Edizione Farmitalia. 535 pp. §
   Emphasizes human medical interrelationships.
291. **CLARENDON, Thomas.** The foot of the horse: its structure and functions, with...a new method of shoeing. **1847**. Dublin: Hodges & Smith. 99 pp. §
   Shoeing based on physiologic principles.

Bracy Clark (1771-1860)

292.__Collected writings. **1815-1859**. London: The author. With numerous plates.
   1. A short history of the horse. **1824**. 56 pp. §
293.__2. Original remarks on the general framing of the horse. **1842**. 20 pp. §
294.__3. Muscles of the posterior extremity of the horse and other domestic quadrupeds. **1842?** 12 pp. §
295.__4. An essay on the bots of horses and other animals. **1815**. 73 pp. §

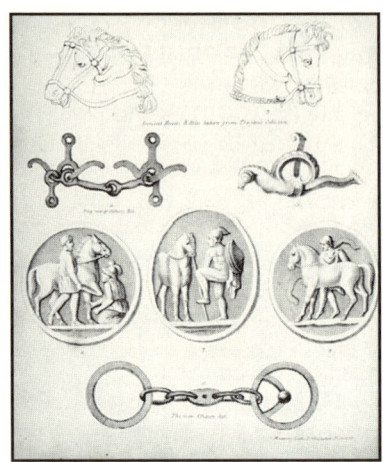

Clark: A treatise on the bits of horses, 1835 (296)

296.__5. A treatise on the bits of horses. **1835**. 2nd ed, 63 pp. §
297.__6. Hippiatria: or the surgery and medicine of horses. **1838**. 50 pp. §
298.__7. On the knowledge of the age of the horse by its teeth. **1826**. 16 pp. §
299.__8. On the usage of the ancients respecting shoeing of the horse. **1831**. 36 pp. §
300.__9. A description of the gripes of horses. **1837**. 28 pp. §
301.__10. The cholera unmasked...causes...mode of treating. **1848**. 17 pp. §
302.__11. Pharmacopoeia equina, or new pharmacopoeia for horses. **1833**. 3rd ed, 52 pp. §
303.__12. On the vices of horses. Condition of horses. **1839**. 42 pp. §
304.__13. Review of Wm Youatt's publication called The Horse. **1854**. 8 pp. §
305.__14. On casting horses for operations. **1842**. 2nd ed, 4 pp. §
306.__15. A short history of the celebrated race-horse, Eclipse. **n.d.** 4 pp. §
307.__16. Description of an economical and useful stove...invented by Bracy Clark. **n.d.** 6 pp. §
308.__17. An exposure of the corruption of the Saxon name Arm's Housen into Alms Houses. **n.d.** 8 pp. §
309.__18. Fragmenta veterinaria, or scraps from my memorandum book. **1859**. 32 pp. §
310.__19. On a new secret powder for horses. **n.d.** 2 pp. §

---

311. **CLARK, James.** First lines of veterinary physiology and pathology. **1806**. Edinburgh: The author. 503 pp.

 A general work, based on human sources.

312.__Observations upon the shoeing of horses: with an anatomical description of the bones of the foot of the horse. Edinburgh: A. Donaldson. **1770**. 62 pp. §

 Sensible writing on shoeing; little on foot.

313.__Observations upon the shoeing of horses: together with ...causes of diseases in the feet of horses... **1775**. Edinburgh: J. Balfour. 204 pp.
  Excellent on shoeing and treatment of foot.
314.__(same) **1782**. Edinburgh: W. Creech. Rev ed, 214 pp.
315.__A treatise on the prevention of diseases incidental to horses from bad management in regard to stables, food, water, air, exercise... **1788** Edinburgh: W. Smellie. 425 pp.
  An enlightened work, even by today's standards.
316.__(same) **1790**. Edinburgh: W. Creech. 427 pp. §
317.__(same) **1791**. Phila: Wm Spotswood. 208 pp. §
318. **CLARKE, J.W.** Cattle problems explained: thirty original essays. **1880**. Battle Creek, MI: The author. 278 pp. §
  On milk yield, breeding, abortion, etc.
319. **CLARKE, William H.** Horses' teeth: a treatise on their mode of development, anatomy, microscopy, pathology, and dentistry. **1886**. New York: J. Reynders. 3rd ed, 292 pp.
  Useful information; with plates on ageing.
320.__(same) **1893**. New York: W.R. Jenkins. 4th ed, 308 pp.
321.__The people's horse, cattle, sheep, and swine doctor...diseases of the respective animals, with exact doses of medicine for each. **1891**. New York: M.T. Richardson. 334 pp. §

Francis Clater (1756-1823)

322.__Every man his own cattle doctor: or, a practical treatise on the diseases of horned cattle... **1810**. London: B. Crosby. 370 pp. §
  Largely unoriginal; promotes sale of remedies.
323.__(same) **1815**. Phila: A. Small. 256 pp.
324.__(same) **1817**. London: Baldwin, Cradock. 5th ed, 392 pp.
  Bound with: Topham: Diseases incident to cattle... (1788) qv.
325.__Every man his own cattle doctor: containing the causes, symptoms and treatment of all the diseases incident to oxen, sheep, swine, poultry, and rabbits. **1836**. London: Baldwin, Cradock. 8th ed, 364 pp.
  Extensively revised, with some improvement.
326.__(same) **1844**. Phila: Lea and Blanchard. 251 pp.
  Rewritten by Youatt and Skinner; much improved.
327.__Every man his own cattle doctor. Entirely rewritten...by George Armatage. **1870?** London: F. Warne; New York: Scribner. 651 pp. §
  A radical revision of Clater's early work.
328.__(same) **1871**. London: F. Warne. 4th ed, Rev, 669 pp. §
329.__Every man his own farrier, or, the whole art of farriery laid open... **1783**. Dublin: Sleater, Moncrieffe. 221 pp.
  Largely from Gibson; unchanged through 20 ed.
330.__(same) **1808**. Newark: A. Tomlinson. 17th ed. 180 pp.
331.__(same) **1809**. London: B. Crosby. 20th ed. 179 pp.
332.__(same) **1810**. 21st ed, Rev, 360 pp.

333.___(same) **1811**. 21st ed, Rev, 360 pp. §
334.___(same) **1817**. London: Baldwin, Cradock. 23rd ed, Rev, 360 pp. §
335.___Every man his own farrier: containing the causes, symptoms, and most approved methods of cure...with a veterinary pharmacopoeia. **1826**. London: Baldwin, Cradock. 25th ed, 379 pp.

   A revision including 74 pp on dogs.

336.___Every man his own farrier: containing the causes, symptoms, and most approved methods of cure of the diseases of horses and dogs. **1843**. London: Cradock & Co. 411 pp.

   A major revision by Edward Mayhew.

337.___Every man his own farrier: containing the causes, symptoms, and most approved methods of cure of the diseases of horses. **1845**. Phila: Lea & Blanchard. 219 pp. §

   First American ed, with notes by J.S. Skinner.

338.___(same as item 336) **1854**. 30th ed, 372 pp. §
339.___Every man his own farrier: containing the mode of treatment and cure of the various diseases incident to...the horse... **1858**. Halifax: Milner & Sowerby. 370 pp.
340.___Clater's every man his own farrier: revised by D. McTaggart: together with: Rarey's treatment and management of the horse. **1860**. Halifax: Milner &: Sowerby. 370 pp. §

   With 64-pp version of Rarey's horse tamer.

341.___(same as item 336) **1861**. London: Longman & Co. 362 pp.
342.___Every man his own horse and cow doctor: with...cause and cure of diseases in sheep. **1870**. London: Milner & Co. 207 pp. §

   Revised by D. McTaggart.

343.(__) Farmers' barn book: containing the causes, symptoms, and treatment of all the diseases incident to oxen, sheep, and swine... **1851**. Phila: W.A. Leary. 311 pp.

   From the "cattle doctor;" additions by Skinner.

---

344. **CLAYTON, G.W.** A treatise on the cat. **1918?** Chicago: [s.n.]. 32 pp.

   A pamphlet promoting the author's remedies.

345. **CLOK, Henry.** The diseases of sheep explained and described, with the proper remedies to prevent and cure the same... **1868**. Phila: Claxton, Ramsen. 146 pp. §

   By a competent veterinarian; well written.

346. **COBBOLD, T(homas) Spencer** (1828-1886). The internal parasites of our domesticated animals... **1873**. London: The Field office. 144 pp. §

   Biology of entozoa of large and small animals.

347. **COBURN, Foster Dwight** (1846-1924). Swine husbandry... management of swine, and the prevention and treatment of their diseases. **1883**. New York: O. Judd. 295 pp.

   A text for agricultural students.

348.___Swine in America: a textbook for the breeder, feeder & student. **1916**. New York: O. Judd. 603 pp. §

   Stresses disease prevention.

349. **COLBY, George.** The horseman's friend, or, pocket counsellor. **1868.** Gettysburg, PA: J.E. Wible. 31 pp.
  A little book of little value.
350. **COLBY, Lucius H.** Care, rearing, and medical treatment of domestic animals. **1875.** Auburn, NY: W.J. Moses. 473 pp.
  Homeopathy, including foot-and-mouth disease.
351. **COLE, Samuel W.** (1796-1851). The American veterinarian...showing the causes, symptoms, and remedies, and rules for restoring and preserving health... **1847.** Boston: J.P. Jewett. 288 pp. §
352.___ **1856.** Boston: J.P. Jewett; Cleveland: Jewett, Proctor. 288 pp. §
353. **(COLEMAN, Edward)** (1765-1839). Observations on the structure, oeconomy, and diseases of the foot of the horse, and on the principles and practice of shoeing. **1798.** Extract from Universal Sportsman, published in Dublin [179?], pp 197-225. §
  "...a collection of crude absurd doctrines...philosophical verbiage..." (Smith)

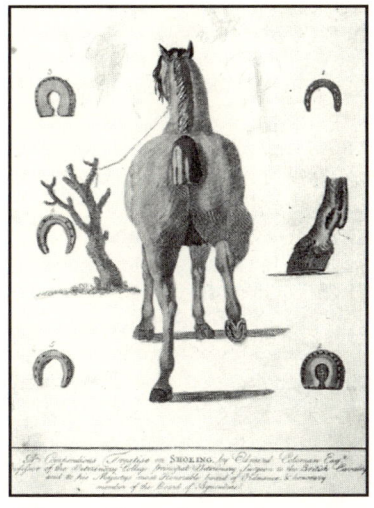

Coleman: Observations on the structure, oeconomy, and diseases of the foot of the horse, 1798 (353)

354. **COLEMAN, Joseph Brine.** Pathological horse-shoeing...theory and practice...also an outline of the anatomy and physiology of the foot of the horse. **1876.** Chicago: H. Fish. 185 pp. §
  A rational system, on physiologic principles.
355. **COLIN, G(abriel)** (1825-1896). Traite de physiologie comparee des animaux...la medecine, zootechnie... **1871-73.** Paris: J.-B. Bailliere. 2 vol, 850; 940 pp. §
  A basic veterinary textbook.

356. **COLUMBRE, Agostino** (fl 1490). I tre libri della natura de I cavalli, et del modo de medicar le loro infermita. **1547.** Vinegia: [s.n.]. 99 pp.
   Good for the time; with anatomy and physiology.
357. **COMPTON, Richard.** A century of caring: One hundred years of organized veterinary medicine in Ohio...1883-1983.**1984.** Columbus: Ohio VMA. 109 pp.
358. **CONN, George H.** The Arabian horse in America. **1957.** Woodstock, NY: Countryman Press. 308 pp. §
   Importation and breeding, from Spanish conquest.
359. **CONRAD, Jack R.** The horn and the sword: the history of the bull as symbol of power and fertility. **1957.** New York: E.P. Dutton. 222 pp. §
360. **CONTE, A.** Jurisprudence veterinaire. **1898.** Paris: J.B. Bailliere. 553 pp.
   Section of French veterinary encyclopedia.
361. **COON, David.** A brief history of dog guides for the blind. **1959.** Morristown, NJ: Seeing Eye. 48 pp. §
   With many informative illustrations.
362. **COOPER, J(ohn) W.** (1803?-). Game fowls, their origin and history...breeds, strains, and crosses. **1869.** West Chester, PA: The author. 304 pp.
   With rules for fighting; section on diseases.
363. **CORNISH, Charles John** (1858-1906). Wild animals in captivity... **1894.** New York: Macmillan. 340 pp.
   Stories of the London zoo; many photos.
364. **COTCHIN, Ernest.** The Royal Veterinary College, London. **1990.** Buckingham: [s.n.]. 232 pp.
   History of the college and British vet med.
365. **COURTENAY, Edward.** Manual of the practice of veterinary medicine. Rev by F.T.G. Hobday. **1906.** New York: W.R. Jenkins. 2nd ed, 573 pp. §
   A long-standard text in Britain and America.
366. __ **1908.** Toronto: J.A. Carveth. 573 pp. §
367. __ The practice of veterinary medicine and surgery. **1894.** Toronto: J.A. Carveth. 589 pp. §
   Based on teaching at Ontario Vet College.
368. **COVINGTON, Nicholas Goza** (1892-). Manual of experimental physiology: practical course... **n.d.** [s.l. s.n.]. 66 pp.
   Lab course for nonphysiology majors.
369. __Manual of physiology: lecture course... **1932.** Ann Arbor, MI: Edwards Bros. 471 pp.
   A basic college textbook.
370. __Manual of practical and experimental pharmacology. **1937.** Pullman, WA: Student Book Corp. 166 pp.
   For use by veterinary students.
371. **COWIE, James.** Reminiscences of the medical and veterinary arts. **1876?** London: [s.n.]. 16 pp.
   By a council member of Royal Vet College.

372. **CRAIG, Robert Alexander** (1872-). Diseases of swine, with special reference to preventive measures... **1906**. New York: O. Judd. 191 pp.
   A brief work for farmers.
373. **CRANE, D.H.** The American horse doctor. **1872**. Holly, MI: [s.n.]. 34 pp. §
   A pamphlet promoting the author's remedies.
374. **CRAWFORD, Andy.** Mules go to war: a tale of floating barns on the high seas during World War II. **1979**. [s.l.]: The author. 87 pp. §
   By a VC remount officer; later AVMA VP.
375. **CROCKER, Walter J.** Veterinary post-mortem technic. **1918**. Phila; London: J.B. Lippincott. 233 pp. §
   An early work on a neglected subject.
376. **CROSS, John** (1790-1850). A history of the variolous epidemic: which occurred in Norwich in the year 1819... **1820**. London: Burgess & Hill. 296 pp.
   History of smallpox and cowpox; vaccination.
377. **CURTICE, Cooper** (1856-1939). The animal parasites of sheep. **1890**. Washington: GPO. 222 pp.
   Descriptive work, with 36 plates.
378. **CUSHING, Harvey** (1869-1939). The life of Sir William Osler. **1940**. London; New York: Oxford Univ Press. 53 + 1417 pp. §
   The definitive biography, incl vet studies.

George H. Dadd (1813-1868)

379.___The advocate of veterinary reform and outlines of anatomy and physiology of the horse... **1850**. Boston: The author. 307 pp. §
   Mediocre, but with extensive vet dictionary.
380.___The American cattle doctor: containing the necessary information for preserving the health and curing the diseases of oxen, cows, sheep, and swine... **1851**. New York: O. Judd. 359 pp. §
   Advocates rational and humane treatment, use of anesthesia (first vet use in America?)
381.___(same) **1856**. New York: C.M. Saxton. 359 pp. §
382.___(same) **1857**. 359 pp. §
383.___(same) **1858**. New York: A.O. Moore. 359 pp, §
384.___(same) **1860**. New York: C.M. Saxton; San Francisco: H.H. Bancroft. 359 pp.
385.___(same) **1864**. New York: C.M. Saxton. 359 pp.
386.___(same) **1865**. New York: O. Judd. 359 pp. §
387.___ The American cattle doctor: a complete work on all the diseases of cattle, sheep, and swine: and...information on the cattle plague and trichina... **1878**. New York: O. Judd; Cincinnati: R.W. Carroll. 367 pp.
   A new work, first published 1869.
388.___(same) **1883**. New York: O. Judd. 367 pp.
389.___(same) **1885**. New York: O. Judd; Cincinnati: R.W. Carroll. 367 pp. §
390.___(same) **1888**. New York: O. Judd. 367 pp.
391.___(same as item 380) **1900**. New York: O. Judd. 359 pp, §
   Introduction by M.C. Weld.

28 *Five Centuries of Veterinary Medicine*

392.__(same) **1907**. 359 pp.
393.__The American reformed cattle doctor... **1851**. Boston: The author. 359 pp. §
    Same content as American cattle doctor (1851).
394.__The American reformed horse book: a treatise on the causes, symptoms, and cure of all the diseases of the horse, including every disease peculiar to America... **1872**. Cincinnati: R.W. Carroll. 442 pp. §
    Urged humane treatment; vet schools in US.
395.__(same) **1878**. New York: O. Judd; Cincinnati: R.W. Caroll. 442 pp.
    First published 1869.
396.__(same) **1883**. New York: O. Judd. 442 pp. §
397.__(same) **1892**. 442 pp.
398.__(same) **1915**. 442 pp.
399.__The anatomy and physiology of the horse...also, a series of examinations on equine anatomy and physiology... **1857**. Boston: J.P. Jewett. 291 pp.
    First such American work; 20 hand-colored plates.
400.__(same) **1859**. New York: A.O. Moore. 291 pp.
    Like 1857 ed, but without colored plates.
401.__(same) **1863**. New York: C.M. Saxton. 291 pp. §
    Like 1857 ed, with 20 hand-colored plates.
402.__Dadd's chart of veterinary reformed practice: being a condensed synopsis of the diseases of horses, cattle and sheep... **1848**. Boston: C. Moody.
    A large folding barn sheet, in board covers.

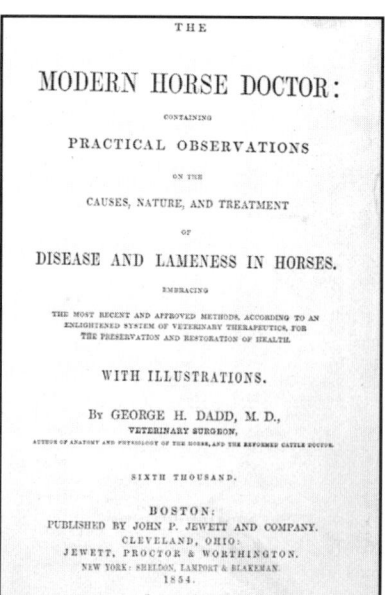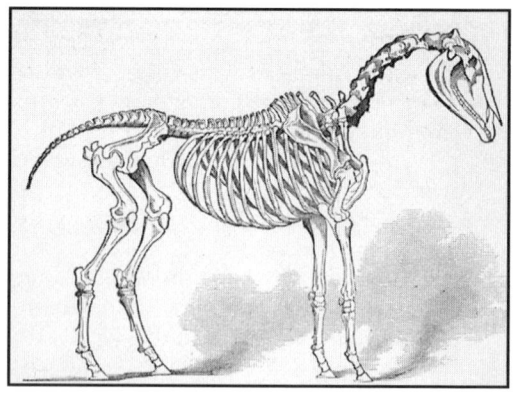

Dadd: 1854 (403)

403.__The modern horse doctor: containing practical observations on the causes, nature, and treatment of disease and lameness in horses... **1854.** Boston: J.P. Jewett. 432 pp. §

    Early advocate of humane and rational treatment by a person (MD) outside the vet profession.

404.__(same) **1855.** 432 pp. §

405.__(same) **1860**, New York: O. Judd. 432 pp.

406.__(same) **1860.** New York: Saxton, Barker; San Francisco: H.H. Bancroft. 432 pp.

407.__(same) **1863.** New York: C.M. Saxton. 432 pp. §

408.__A practical treatise on the most obvious diseases peculiar to horses, together with directions for their most rational treatment... **1865.** Chicago: Lord & Smith; New York: Blakeman & Mason. 142 pp.

    Includes section on art of shoeing.

---

409. **DALE-GREEN, Patricia.** Cult of the cat. 1963. New York: Weathervane Books. **1898.** 189 pp. §

    The cat in mythology, superstition and magic.

410. **DALRYMPLE, W(illiam) H(addock)** (1856-1925). Livestock sanitation... **1923.** Baton Rouge, LA: Gladney Press. 145 pp. §

    A collection of short popular articles.

411. **DALZIEL, Hugh.** British dogs...history, characteristics, breeding, management, and exhibition... **1895?** London: L. Upcott Gill. 2 vol, 2nd ed. 503; 526 pp. §

    Details of breeds, numerous plates.

412.__Diseases of dogs: their causes, symptoms, and treatment...and brief directions for maintaining a dog in health. **1905.** London: L. Upcott Gill; New York: Scribner's. 4th ed, 142 pp. §

    A brief work for owners.

413.__The diseases of horses: their pathology, diagnosis and treatment... **1900?** London: L. Upcott Gill. 102 pp. §

    A handbook in dictionary form for owners.

414. **DANFORTH, Alonzo H.** (1837-). The science of practical horsemanship...with a description of its diseases and treatment... **1869.** Montpelier, VT: Argus & Patriot. 248 pp. §

415. **DANIEL, William Barker** (1753?-1833). Rural sports. **1801.** London: Bunny & Gold. 3 vol, 378; 535; 356 pp. §

    On dogs, hunting, fishing, birds; fine plates.

416.__Supplement to the rural sports. **1813.** London: B. & R. Crosby. 742 pp. §

417. **DANIELS, A.C.** Diseases of the dog: the dog doctor. **1911.** Boston: The author. 62 pp. §

    Proprietary remedies for home treatment.

418. **DASSY, Abel.** Le remede a cote du mal. Les maladies des petits animaux domestiques... **1923.** Paris: Librairie Speciale Agricole. 97 pp. §

    Diseases and treatment of small animals.

419. **DAVENPORT, E(ugene)** (1856-1941). Principles of breeding...economic improvement of domesticated animals and plants. **1907**. Boston: Ginn. 727 pp. §
    A basic textbook of applied genetics.

420. **DAY, SON & HEWITT.** The half-crown key to farriery... **1869**. London: W. Kent. 147 pp. §
    A mediocre work promoting authors' remedies.

421. **de GREY, Thomas.** The compleat horse-man and expert ferrier...the best manner of breeding good horses...how to know and cure all maladies and diseases in horses... **1639**. London: T. Harper. 356 pp.
    Largely unoriginal, but urges study of animal disease by educated men.

422. __(same) **1670**. 4th ed, 583 pp. §

423. **De VINE, J(ohn) F(rancis)** (1874-). Bovine tuberculosis...with [additions by] E.Z. Russell...D.F. Luckey...O.E. Dyson. **1917**. Chicago: Am Vet Publ Co. 120 pp.
    On prevalence and control of bovine TB.

424. **DIEGENDESCH, Johannes.** Nachrichters nutzliches und aufrichtiges Ross-artzney-buchlein... **1770**. Basel: [s.n.]. 223 pp.
    Treatment of horse and cattle diseases.

425. __Nachrichters nutzliches und aufrichtiges Pferd-artzneybuch... **1822**. Harrisburg, PA: J.S. Wiestling. 216 pp.
    A Pennsylvania German version of the 1770 ed.

426. **DELAFOND, O.** Traite de pathologie generale comparee des animaux domestiques. **1855**. Paris: Labe. 2nd ed, 724 pp. §
    Symptoms and lesions given by body systems.

427. **DELISSER, George P.** Delisser's horsemans' guide: comprising the laws on warranty and the rules in purchasing and selling horses... **1875**. New York: Dick & Fitzgerald. 90 pp. §
    How to determine age and soundness.

428. **DEMAREE, Albert Lowther** (1894-). The American agricultural press, 1819-1860. **1941**. New York: Columbia Univ Press. 430 pp. §
    The early farm journals; items of vet interest.

429. **DENHARDT, Robert M.** The horse of the Americas. **1947**. Norman, OK: Univ Okla Press. 286 pp. §
    Role of the western horse in US history; with 5 related articles from Spanish-Barb Quarterly.

430. __(same) **1975**. Rev ed, paperback, 343 pp. §
    A substantial revision of the first edition.

431. **DICK, William** (1793-1866). Manual of veterinary science. **1862**. Edinburgh: A. & C. Black. 104 pp. §
    Prepared as article for Encyclopaedia Britannica.

432. __Occasional papers on veterinary subjects...with a memoir by R.O. Pringle. **1869**. Edinburgh and London: W. Blackwood. 501 pp.
    Contains 45 papers and posthumous biography.

Dictionaries

433.__BEGIN, L(ouis) J(acques) (1793-1859). Dictionaire des termes de medecine, chirurgie, anatomie, art veterinaire, pharmacie...etc. **1830**. Paris: J.B. Bailliere. 619 pp. §
   An early dictionary including vet medicine.

434.__BOARDMAN, Thomas. A dictionary of the veterinary art. **1805**. London: G. Kearsley. §
   A large work (unpaged) by an educated man.

435.__BUC'HOZ, Pierre-Joseph (1731-1807) Dictionaire veterinaire et des animaux domestiques. **1775**. Paris: Brunet. Vol 6 (of 6), 175 pp. §
   Bound with: Fauna Gallicus, listing 779 animal species common to France; bibliographies.

436.__COOPER, Samuel (1780-1848). A dictionary of practical surgery...an account of the instruments, remedies, and applications employed in surgery. **1822**. New York: Collins and Hannay. From 4th London ed. Vol 1, 704 pp. §
   Encyclopedic style; Abdomen—Hemorrhoids.

437.__The complete English farmer, or a general dictionary of husbandry. **1766**. London: G. Cooke
   Includes diseases of horses and cattle.

438.__COXE, John R. The Philadelphia medical dictionary...containing all the terms used in medicine, surgery, pharmacy...and materia medica. **1838**. Phila: T. Dobson. 2nd ed, 433 pp. §
   Mainly terms of Latin origin; brief definitions.

439.__DEANE, Samuel (1733-1814). The New-England farmer: or, Georgical dictionary... **1790**. Worcester: I. Thomas. 335 pp. §
   Entries on diseases of domestic animals.

440.__(same) **1822**. Boston: Wells and Lilly. 3rd ed, 532 pp. §

441.__Dictionarium rusticum, urbanicum & botanicum: or, a dictionary of husbandry...[etc]. **1726**. London: J. & J. Knapton. 2 vol. Unpaged. §
   Entries on farriery, riding, cattle diseases.

442.__DUNGLISON, Robley (1798-1869). A dictionary of medical sciences: containing...terms of anatomy, physiology, pathology [etc]. **1874**. Phila: H.C. Lea. Rev ed, 1131 pp. §
   A classic American work; numerous editions.

443.__ __Medical lexicon. A dictionary of medical science... **1857**. Phila: Blanchard & Lea. 15th ed, 992 pp. §

444.__(same) **1866**. Phila: H.C. Lea. Rev ed, 1047 pp. §

445.__The farrier's and horseman's dictionary: being a complete system of horsemanship. **1726**. London: J. Darby. 454 pp.

446.__HOBLYN, Richard Dennis (1803-1886). A dictionary of terms used in medicine and the collateral sciences. **1835**. London: Sherwood, Gilbert. 328 pp. §
   Some veterinary terms; quack medicine section.

447.__ __(same) **1846**. Phila: Lea & Blanchard. 1st American ed, from 2nd English, 402 pp. §

448.__HOOPER, R. A new medical dictionary. 1817. Phila: B. Warner, M. Carey. 870 pp. §
   Based on Quincy's Lexicon-Medicum.
449.__HUNTER, James. A complete dictionary of farriery & horsemanship: containing the art of farriery... 1796. Dublin: Wogan, P. Byrne. Unpaged.
   A mediocre work; useful for identifying terms.
450.__HURTREL D'ARBOVAL, L.H.J. Dictionaire de medecine, de chirurgie et d'hygiene veterinaire. 1874. Paris: J.B. Bailliere. 3 vol, 1004; 974; 926 pp. §
   An encyclopedic work with many text figures.
451.__MERIC, Henry Eugene de (1849-). Dictionary of medical terms: English-French. 1899. London: Bailliere, Tindall. 394 pp. §
452.__QUAIN, Richard, Sir (1816-1898). A dictionary of medicine: including general pathology, general therapeutics, hygiene, and the diseases peculiar to women and children. 1883. New York: D. Appleton. 1816 pp. §
453.__THOMAS, Joseph (1811-1891). A complete pronouncing medical dictionary...with signification, etymology, and pronunciation. 1887. Phila: J.B. Lippincott. 844 pp. §
454.__ __A comprehensive medical dictionary: containing the pronunciation, etymology, and significance of the terms... 1875. Phila: J.B. Lippincott. 704 pp. §
   Includes a materia medica.
455.__WALLIS, Thomas. The farrier's and horseman's complete dictionary. 1775. London: Longmans, Green. 3rd ed, unpaged.
   Good synopsis of contemporary practice.

---

456. DIGHTON, Charles Allen Adair. The bull-terrier and all about it. 1920. Manchester: Our Dogs Publ Co. 57 pp.
   Breeding, management and showing of the breed.
457. DIMOCK, W.W.; EDWARDS, P.R. Hemolytic streptococci of horses and other animals... 1933. Lexington: Kentucky AES Bull 338. 53 pp.
458. DIMSDALE, Thomas (1712-1800). Tracts on inoculation... observations on epidemic smallpox... 1781. London: W. Owen. 248 pp.
   Introduction of inoculation in Russia.
   DINKS, MAYHEW & HUTCHISON—see W.H. Herbert.
459. DIOSCORIDES PEDANIUS, of Anazarbos (fl 60 AD). Dioscoride fatto di greco italiano...per la materia medesima. 1542. Venetia: Curtio Troiano adi Navo. 311 pp. §
   Italian trans of classic 1stC materia medica.
460. DOBIE, J(ames) Frank (1888-1964). The longhorns. 1941. Boston: Little, Brown. 388 pp.
   A classic work on the subject.
461. (DOGS). Hints to dog owners: a manual for the daily use of dog owners. breeders...& others in the care and treatment of dogs. 1927. London: A.F. Shirley. 143 pp.
   A brief work promoting canine remedies.

462. **DOLLAR, John Archibald Watt.** A handbook of horse-shoeing...anatomy and physiology of the horse's foot. **1898.** New York: W.R. Jenkins. 438 pp.
  Normal and pathologic shoeing related to structure and function; many illustrations.
463.__The practice of veterinary surgery. **1908.** New York: W.R. Jenkins. Vol 1, 265 pp. §
  Includes restraint, anesthesia, antisepsis, wounds, castration; J.V. Lacroix signature.
464.__Regional veterinary surgery and operative technique... **1912.** Toronto: J.F. Hartz. 1131 pp.
  Copiously illustrated; E.A. Ehmer signature.
465. (__) Dollar's veterinary surgery: general, operative, and regional. **1952.** London: Bailliere, Tindall. 1036 pp.
  A major revision by J.J. O'Connor.
466. **DOUGLAS, James** (1675-1742). Myographiae comparatae specimen, or, a comparative description of all the muscles in a man, and in a quadruped... **1760.** Edinburgh: A. Kincaid & J. Bell. 219 pp. §
  Includes "the muscles peculiar to a woman."
467. **DOWNING, Joseph.** A treatise on the disorders incident to horned cattle...their symptoms, and the most rational methods of cure. **1815.** Kidderminster: G. Gower. 95 pp.
  Plagiarizes Topham (qv), but with excellent original appendix on extraction of calves.
468.__(same) **1813.** Phila: A. Finley. 145 pp. §
469. **Du HUYS, Charles.** The Percheron horse. **1868.** New York: O. Judd. 100 pp. §
  Breeding and characteristics of Percherons.
470. **DUN, Finley** (1830-1897). Veterinary medicines: their actions and uses. **1854.** Edinburgh: Sutherland & Knox. 598 pp.
  An extensive materia medica and pharmacopoeia.
471.__(same) **1859.** 520 pp.
472.__(same) **1882.** New York: W.R. Jenkins. 598 pp. §
473.__(same) **1883.** 598 pp. §
474.__(same) **1886.** 598 pp. §
475.__(same) **1900.** 9th ed, 776 pp.
476. **DUNBAR, Alexander.** A treatise on the diseases incident to the horse, especially those of the foot... **1873.** Wilmington, DE: James & Webb. 240 pp. §
  Eccentric system for treating contracted hooves.
477. **DUNCAN, A.** The Edinburgh new dispensatory. **1806.** Edinburgh: Bell & Bradfute. 762 pp. §
  Includes London (1791) and Dublin (1794) editions.
478. **DUNNINGTON, John C., & Son.** The horseman's friend: giving the causes and symptoms of diseases the horse is subject to... **1884.** Peoria: IL: J.W. Franks. 111 pp.
  Simplistic: "a child of ten years can understand."

479. **DUVAL, Mathias** (1844-1907). Cours de physiologie... **1879**. Paris: J.B. Bailliere. 758 pp. §
   An elementary human physiology text.
480. **DWYER, Francis**. On seats and saddles, bits and bitting and the prevention and cure of restiveness in horses. **1869**. Phila: Lippincott. 255 pp.
   A work on riding and control of horses.
481. **DYKSTRA, Ralph R.** (1879-1962). Veterinary medicine in Kansas. **1954**. Manhattan, KS: [s.n.]. 110 pp. §
   History of Kansas VMA; biographies of pioneers.
482. **EBERLEIN, Richard Karl** (1859-). Die Hufkrankheiten des Pferdes... **1908**. Wien; Leipzig: W. Praumuller. 560 pp. §
   Details of hoof diseases; early radiographs.
483. **EDELMANN, Richard; MOHLER, John R.; EICHORN, A.** Meat hygiene. **1919**. Phila: Lea & Febiger. 4th ed, 472 pp. §
   From classic German work; E.R. Frank signature.
484. **EHRENFELS, Joseph Michael** (1767-1843). Erdmann Hulfreichs unterricht fur Bauersleute von den Krankheiten der Pferde, des Hornviehs... **1793**. Wien: A. Doll. 181 pp. §
   Diseases of horses, cattle, sheep and swine.
485. **(ELEPHANT)**. Burmese elephant medicines. **1890**. Rangoon: British Burma Press. 43 pp.
   History of elephant medicine; English, Burmese.
486. **ELLENBERGER, Wilhelm** (1848-1929). Grundriss der vergleichenden Histologie der Haussaugethier. **1888**. Berlin: P. Parey. 270 pp.
   An early text on histology of domestic animals.
487.__Histologie der Haussaugethiere fur Thierartze und Studierende. **1884**. Berlin: P. Parey. Part 1, 308 pp.
   Written for veterinarians and students.
488.__Lehrbuch der allgemeinen Therapie des Haussaugethiere. **1885**. Berlin: Hirschwald. 724 pp.
   A handbook of therapy for farm animals.
489.__; **BAUM, Hermann** (1854-1932). Anatomie descriptive et topographique du chien. **1894**. Paris: C. Reinwald. 640 pp. §
   Detailed canine anatomy; trans from German.
490. **ELLWOOD, Guilford S.** A partial history of the Chicago Veterinary Medical Association. **1966**. [s.l. s.n.]. 81 pp. §
   With details of monthly meetings, 1916-1944.
491. **ERK, Nihal.** XVIence asir veteriner...eserler. **1955**. Ankara: Yeni Desen Matbaasi. 65 pp. §
   A study of 16thC vet med in Turkey.
492. **EVANS, Anna Margaret** (1914); **BARKER, C(lifford) A(lbert) V(ictor)** (1919-). Century one: a history of the Ontario Veterinary Association, 1874-1974. **1976**. Guelph, Ont: A.M. Evans. 516 pp. §
   Details of association matters, legal documents.

493. **EVANS, Guerdon**. The dairyman's manual: being a complete guide for the American dairyman. **1851**. Utica, NY: J.W. Fuller. 235 pp. §
Includes sections on treatment of diseases.

494. **EWART, J(ames) C(ossar)** (1851-1933). A critical period in the development of the horse. **1897**. London: A. & C. Black. 27 pp. §
Observations on early embryology of the horse.

495. **FABRICIUS, ab Aquapendente** (ca 1533-1619). The embryological treatises of Hieronymus Fabricius of Aquapendente: the formation of the egg and of the chick. The formed fetus. **1941**. Ithaca, NY: Cornell Univ Press. Facsimile 1621 ed; trans and commentary by H.B. Adelmann. 2 vol, 376; 266 pp.
The definitive translation of this classic.

496.__(same) **1942**. 2 vol, 833 pp. §

497. **FANTUS, Bernard** (1874-).The technic of medication...methods of prescribing and preparation... **1926**. Chicago: AMA Press. 335 pp.
For physicians, but with veterinary applications.

Farriery

498.__The complete farrier and horse doctor: the habits, diseases, and management of the horse... **1850**. New York: Dewitt & Davenport. New ed, 126 pp. §
A handbook with emphasis on management.

499.__The complete farrier, or, gentleman's travelling companion... **1809**. Phila: Bradford & Inskeep. 248 pp.
Pulse in diagnosis; maintenance of health.

500.__The domestic animal's friend: or, the complete Virginia and Maryland farrier... **1818**. Winchester, VA: J. Foster. 436 pp.
A typical "farrier," but with extracts from Clark's work on prevention of disease.

501.__Ein newe und bewerte Rossartzney... **1583**. Strassburg: N. Wyriot. 170 pp.
Equine diseases; includes "der Wolff" in tail.

502.__Every man his own farrier and cattle doctor...diseases of horses, horned cattle and sheep. **1916**. Plymouth: W. Brendon. 305 pp. §
In the tradition of Clater; many recipes.

503.__The farmer's and horseman's true guide...with useful recipes. **1834**. Owego, NY: A.P. Searing. 132 pp. §
An ordinary work, typical of the time.

504.__The farmer's receipt book and pocket farrier: being a choice selection of...receipts... **1831**. Concord, NH: Fisk & Chase. 214 pp.
A mediocre work, mainly from British sources.

505.__The gentleman and farmer's general book of knowledge, etc. **1795**. Ripon: W. Darnton. 168 pp. §
A compilation of worthless cures (British).

506.__The new American pocket farrier and farmer's guide in the choice and management of horses, neat cattle, sheep and swine... **1845**. Phila: J.B. Perry. 284 pp.
A mediocre work, largely British sources.

36   *Five Centuries of Veterinary Medicine*

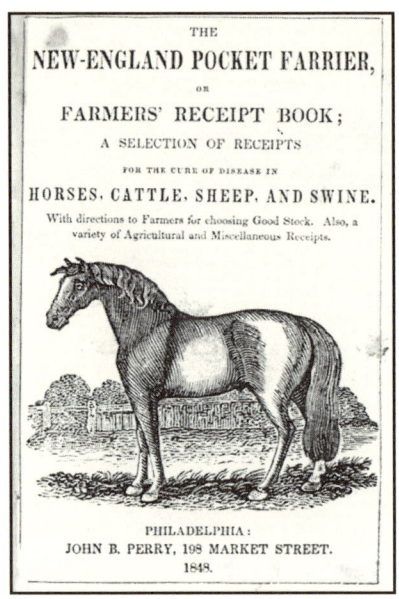

Anon: 1848 (507)

507.__The New-England pocket farrier, or, farmer's receipt book... **1848**. Phila: J.B. Perry. 214 pp. §
   Identical to item 509.
508.__The pocket-farrier, or, approved receipts...to cure or assist in...accidents that may happen to a horse... **1778**. Shrewsbury: W. Williams. 35 pp. §
   A tiny book of remedies, some in old handwriting.
509.__The pocket farrier, or, farmer's receipt book...for the cure of disease in horses, cattle, sheep, and swine... **1836**. Boston: C. Gaylord. 214 pp. §
   A mediocre work from various sources.
510.__The practical farrier...containing rules for breeding and training of colts... **1737**. London: T. Longman & T. Astley. 112 pp.
   An ordinary work like many others of its kind.

---

511. **FAVILLE, George C.** The Virginia State Veterinary Medical Association. **1931**. Richmond: [s.n.]. 70 pp. §
   History 1894-1931, with author reminiscences.
512. **FELDMAN, William H(ugh)** (1892-). Neoplasms of domesticated animals... **1932**. Phila; London: W.B. Saunders. 410 pp. §
   An early work, by a noted veterinary pathologist.
513. **FELIZET, Charles Laurent.** Dictionaire veterinaire: hygiene, medecine, chirurgie, pharmacie... **1883**. Paris: J. Rothschild. 452 pp.
   In miniature encyclopedia format.
514. **FERON, John.** A new system of farriery: including...external structure of the horse...improved mode of treatment... **1803**. London: J. Johnson. 272 pp.
   Promotes methods of the London school.

515. **FESSENDEN, Thomas Green** (1771-1837). Moubray on breeding, rearing and fattening all kinds of...domestic animals. **1837.** Boston: J. Breck; New York: G.C. Thorburn. 2nd American ed. 278 pp. §
   A brief work on poultry and animal husbandry.
516. **FIELD, John.** Posthumous extracts from the veterinary records of the late John Field. Edited by his brother, William Field. **1843.** London: Longman, Brown. 236 pp.
   Reports of acute cases by a careful observer.
517. **FISH, Pierre Augustine** (1865-1931). Book of veterinary doses, therapeutic terms and prescription writing. **1919.** Ithaca, NY: Comstock Publ Co. 185 pp.
   Mainly a handbook of materia medica.
518.__Practical exercises in comparative physiology and urine analysis. **1898.** Ithaca, NY: Andrus & Church. 71 pp. §
   Laboratory guide for veterinary students.
519.__Practical exercises in comparative physiology: Part 2. **1901.** Ithaca, NY: Ithaca Jnl Press. 130 pp. §
520. **FITZWYGRAM, Frederick Wellington John, Sir.** (1832-1904). Horses and stables. **1894.** London: Longmans, Green. 4th ed. 560 pp. §
   Disease treatment; curious ideas on contagion.
521.__(same) **1901.** 5th ed, 560 pp.
522.__Notes on shoeing horses. **1863.** London: Smith, Elder. 2nd ed, 127 pp. §
   Includes structure and diseases of the foot.

George Fleming (1833-1901)

523.__Animal plagues: their history, nature, and prevention. **1871.** London: Chapman & Hall. 548 pp. §
   An exhaustive history from early times to 1800.
524.__Horse-shoes and horse-shoeing: their origin, history, uses, and abuses. **1869.** London: Chapman & Hall. 642 pp. §
   A comprehensive history from earliest times.
525.__Human and animal variolae: a study in comparative pathology. **1881.** London: Bailliere, Tindall. 61 pp.
   Prevalence of animal poxes; human vaccination.
526.__A manual of veterinary sanitary science and police... **1875.** London: Chapman & Hall. 2 vol, 561; 660 pp. §
   An early work on veterinary public health.
527.__The practical horse keeper. **1890.** London: L. Upcott Gill. 269 pp. §
   A useful work for owners.
528.__Practical horseshoeing. **1872.** New York: D. Appleton. 108 pp. §
529.__(same) **1872.** New York: W.R. Jenkins. 108 pp. §
530.__Rabies and hydrophobia: their history, nature, causes, symptoms, and prevention. **1872.** London: Chapman & Hall. 405 pp. §
   An extensive history, including treatment.

531.__Roaring in horses (laryngismus paralyticus): its history, nature, causes, prevention, and treatment. **1889**. London: Bailliere, Tindall; New York: W.R. Jenkins. 160 pp.

532.__A text-book of operative veterinary surgery. **1884**. London: Bailliere, Tindall; New York: W.R. Jenkins. Vol 1, 266 pp. §

533.__(same) **1884**. London; New York; Toronto: Williamson & Co. Vol 1, 266 pp. §

A long-time standard text; many illustrations.

534.__A text-book of veterinary obstetrics: including the diseases and accidents incidental to pregnancy... **1889**. New York: W.R. Jenkins. 773 pp. §

A classic work with many illustrations.

535.__(same) **1891**. 773 pp.

536.__(same) **1898**. 2nd ed, 758 pp.

537.__(same) **1907**. 758 pp.

538.__(same) **1908**. 758 pp.

539. (__) Fleming's text-book of operative veterinary surgery. Rev by J. MacQueen. **1903**. London: Bailliere, Tindall. 2nd ed, 696 pp. §

General and special surgery; 2 vol in one.

540. (__) Fleming's veterinary obstetrics... Rev by J.F. Craig. **1912**. London: Bailliere, Tindall. 3rd ed, 528 pp.

An abridged version of earlier editions.

541. (__) (same) **1916**. Chicago: A. Eger. 528 pp. §

542. (__) (same) **1930**. 4th ed, 552 pp. §

543. (__) Lectures on veterinary obstetrical work...training on the delivery of colts, calves, lambs, pigs and dogs... **1903**. Detroit: Detroit Vet...Supply. 280 pp. §

A pirated abridgement of Fleming's obstetrics.

---

544. **FLEXNER, Simon** (1863-1946); **FLEXNER, James T.** William Henry Welch and the heroic age of American medicine. **1941**. New York: Viking Press. 539 pp. §

Includes his work on hog cholera and public health.

545. **FLIGHT, Edward G.** The true legend of St Dunstan and the devil. **1871**. London: Bell & Daldy. 64 pp. §

The horseshoe as a charm against witchcraft.

546. **FLINT, Charles Louis** (1824-1829). Milch cows and dairy farming: comprising the breeds, breeding, and management, in health and disease... **1859**. Boston: A. Williams. 416 pp. §

A general text; short section on disease.

547.__(same) **1860**. Boston: Crosby, Nichols. New ed, 426 pp. §

Gives symptoms and treatment of pleuropneumonia.

548. **FORGRAVE, B.T.G.** A history of the Royal Army Veterinary Corps. **1987**. [s.l. s.n.]. 17 pp. §

Development of RAVC, 1796-1982.

549. **FORREST, Christopher.** The complete American farrier, and horse doctor... **1870**. London: W. Nicholson. 335 pp. §

Typical of its time; includes Dr Chase's recipes.

550.__(same) **1870**. Wakefield: W. Nicholson. 335 pp. §

551.__De Witt's complete American farrier and horse doctor... **1870**. New York: R.M. De Witt. 208 pp.

Essentially like the British edition.

FORRESTER, Frank—see H.W. Herbert

552. **FOX, Claire Gilbride.** The Fairman Rogers collection on the horse and equitation: a history and guide. **1975**. Phila: College of Physicians. 177 pp. §

A catalog of 868 items, many of vet interest.

553. **FRAISSE, E.-C.** Le cheval: organisation, conformation exterieure... production et elevage. **1927**. Paris: Librairie Hachette. 268 pp. §

Equine husbandry, including care of feet.

554. **FRANCK, Ludwig** (1834-1884). Handbuch der tierarztlichen Geburtshilfe. **1887**. Berlin: P. Parey. 2nd ed, rev by Ph. Goring, 740 pp.

A textbook of veterinary obstetrics.

555. **FRANKLIN, Augustus.** The American farrier...being a sure guide to prevent and cure all maladies that are incident to horses...[and] cattle. **1803**. Strasburg, (PA?): Brown & Bowman. 290 pp.

A retrograde work with nasty & brutal remedies.

556. **FREEMAN, Strickland.** The art of horsemanship. **1806**. London: The author. 254 pp.

Riding system like that of Duke of Newcastle.

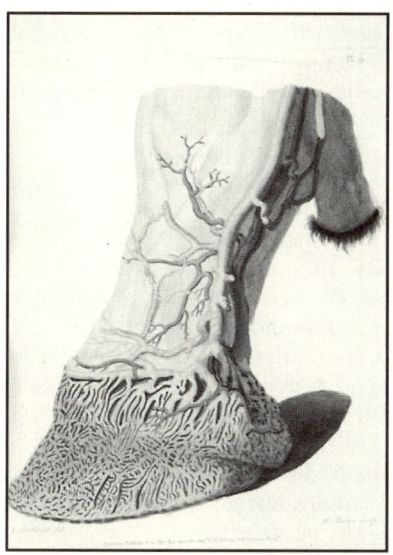

Freeman: Observations on the mechanism of the horse's foot, 1796 (557)

557.__Observations on the mechanism of the horse's foot: its natural spring explained, and a mode of shoeing recommended... **1796**. London: The author. 107 pp.

A remarkably original work by a layman.

558. **FRENCH, Cecil.** Surgical diseases and surgery of the dog. **1906.** Washington: The author. 408 pp. §
An early authoritative work on the subject.
559. **FRICK, Hermann.** Outline of the antiseptic treatment of wounds: for veterinarians. Trans by A. Eger. **1900.** Chicago: A. Eger. 114 pp. §
An early work on wound disinfection.
560. **FRIEDBERGER, Franz** (1839-1902); **FROHNER, Eugene** (1858-1940). Pathology and therapeutics of the domestic animals. Trans by W.L. Zuill. **1895.** Phila: W.L. Zuill. 2 vol, 598; 676 pp. §
A classic work trans from German & French.
561. (__) Friedberger & Frohner's veterinary pathology. Trans by M.H. Hayes. **1904.** London: Hurst & Blackett; Chicago: W.T. Keener. 2 vol, 4th ed, 519; 767 pp.
With translator's signature.
562. (__) (same) **1908.** 2 vol, 6th ed, 731; 702 pp.
563. (__) (same) **1909.** Chicago: Chicago Medical Book Co. 2 vol, 6th ed, 731; 702 pp. §
564. (__) (same) **1910.** London: Hurst & Blackett. 6th ed. §
J.V. Lacroix signature in both volumes.
565. **FRIEDMAN, Reuben.** Biology of Acarus scabiei. **1942.** New York: Froben Press. 183 pp. §
Historical survey (100-p) of 17th-19thC work.
566. **FROHNER, Eugene.** Arzneiverordnungslehre fur...thierarztlich-chemische Untersuchungsmethoden. **1890.** Stuttgart: Ferdinand Enke. 334 pp.
A veterinary materia medica and pharmacopoeia.
567.__Lehrbuch der Arzneimittellehre fur Thierarzte. **1896.** Stuttgart: F. Enke. 608 pp.
Materia medica and pharmacopoeia, revised.
568.__General surgery. Trans by D.H. Udall. **1906.** Ithaca, NY: Taylor & Carpenter. 322 pp. §
From 3rd revised German edition.
569.__(same) **1918.** New York: Macmillan. 347 pp. §
570.__Text-book of general therapeutics for veterinarians. Trans by L.A. Klein. **1916.** Phila; London: J.B. Lippincott. 309 pp.
An excellent text; from 4th German edition.
571. **FUSSELL, G(eorge) E(dwin)** (1889-). More old English farming books from Tull to the Board of Agriculture, 1731-1793. **1950.** London: C. Lockwood. 186 pp. §
Includes several books of veterinary interest.
572.__The old English farming books from Fitzherbert to Tull, 1523-1730. **1947.** London: C Lockwood. 141 pp. §
Numerous works of veterinary interest.
573. **FUSSNECKER, John; AMA, Wilhelm.** Der Thierarzt... Goldenes Hausbuch fur Farmer, Gartner, Pferde- und Viehbesitzer. **1875.** Milwaukee: Herold. 227 pp.
A handbook on animal disease; German-American.

574. **GALVAYNE, Sydney.** Horse dentition: showing how to tell exactly the age of a horse up to thirty years. **1887?** Glasgow: T. Murray. 2nd ed, 25 pp + plates. §
   A copiously illustrated, accurate work.
575. **GAMBADO, Geoffrey** (pseud Henry Bunbury). An academy for grown horsemen. **1787.** London: W. Dickinson. 38 pp. §
   A satire on customs; with 10 amusing plates.
576. __(same) **1905.** Reprint, 120 pp. §
   In small format, with color plates.
577. **GAMGEE, John** (1831-1894). The cattle plague: with official reports of the International Veterinary Congresses, held in Hamburg, 1863, and in Vienna, 1865. **1866.** London: R. Hardwicke. 859 pp. §
   An exhaustive work by an eminent authority.
578. __Diseased meat sold in Edinburgh, and meat inspection, in connection with the public health... **1857.** Edinburgh: Sutherland & Knox. 32 pp.
   Decries the traffic in diseased meat.
579. __Our domestic animals in health and disease. **1861.** London: A. Fullarton. 2 vol, 631; 640 pp.
   A basic work on anatomy and physiology.
580. __(same) **1861-64.** Edinburgh: Thomas C. Jack. 2 vol in 4, 256; 384; 320; 311 pp.
581. __(same) **1865.** Edinburgh: A. Fullarton. Part 3 only, 320 pp. §
582. **GAMGEE, Joseph Sampson** (1828-1886). The cattle plague and diseased meat, in their relations with the public health... **1857.** London: T. Richards. 41 pp.
   A protest against rinderpest in meat animals.
583. __(same) ...A second letter to the Rt. Hon. Sir George Grey... **1857.** 26 pp.
584. **GARBUTT, Raymond J.** Diseases and surgery of the dog, alphabetically arranged. **1938.** New York: O. Judd. 332 pp. Author's signature.
585. __(same) **1948.** 332 pp.
586. **GARCIA CAVERO, Francisco.** Institutiones de albeyteria, y examen de practicantes de ella... **1804.** Madrid: Ramon Ruiz. 62 pp.
   A quiz compend on veterinary medicine.
587. **GARCIA CONDE, Pedro.** Verdadera albeyteria...en qvarto libros...delineadas las enfermedades que sobrevienen en el cuerpo, bracos, y piernas del cavallo... **1707.** Madrid: A. Conçalez. 394 pp.
   On anatomy and diseases of the horse.
588. **GARDENIER, Andrew A.** (ed). Hand-book of ready reference. **1897.** Springfield, MA: King-Richardson. 636 pp. §
   An encyclopedic work for stock owners.
589. __The successful stockman and manual of husbandry. **1899.** Springfield, MA: King-Richardson. 636 pp. §
   Like item 588; folding manikins of horse & cow.
590. **GARRARD, Kenner.** Nolan's system for training cavalry horses. **1862.** New York: D. Van Nostrand. 162 pp. §
   French system adapted to US Army.

591. **GARRISON, Fielding H(udson)** (1870-1933). An introduction to the history of medicine, with medical chronology... **1921**. Phila; London: W.B. Saunders. 3rd ed, 942 pp. §

   A classic work, with few references to vet med.
592. __(same) **1924**. 942 pp.
593. **GARSAULT, Francois A(lexandre) de** (1692-1788?). Le nouveau parfait marechal, ou, la connoissance generale et universelle du cheval... **1770**. Paris: Chez le Clerc. 4th ed, 641 pp. §

   Management, diseases and surgery of the horse.
594. **GARZONI, Marino** (fl 1688-1692). L'arte di ben conoscere, e distinguere le qualita de' cavalli... **1733**. Venezia: Andrea Poletti. 4th ed, 403 pp.

   Includes internal and external diseases of horse.
595. **GATTINGER, Friston Eugene** (1921-). A century of challenge: a history of the Ontario Veterinary College. **1962**. Toronto: Univ Toronto Press. 224 pp. §

   Presented in epochs based on principalships.
596. **GENGA, Bernardino** (1636?-1734?). Anatomy improved and illustrated with regard to...bones and muscles of the human body... **1971?** New York: Editions Medicina Rara. Facsimile 1723 ed, 58 pp. §

   From the London ed; with 42 exquisite plates.
597. **GEORGE, Henry**. A compendious history of the small-pox: with an account of a mode of local treatment... **1833**. London: J. Churchill. 112 pp.

   From 10thC BC, with little on vaccination.
598. **GERSDORFF, Hans von** (-1529). Feldtbuch der Wundtarztney. **1971?** New York: Editions Medicina Rara. Facsimile 1517 ed, unpaged. §

   Wound surgery; from the Strassbourg edition.

William Gibson (1680?-1750)

599. __The farrier's dispensatory...containing a description of the medicinal simples, commonly made use of in the diseases of horses... **1721**. London: W. Taylor. 306 pp.

   The first veterinary pharmacopoeia in English.
600. __(same) **1726**. London: J. Osborn & T. Longman. 2nd ed, 306 pp.
601. __(same) **1734**. London: T. Longman. 4th ed, 306 pp. §
602. __(same) **1741**. 5th ed, 306 pp.

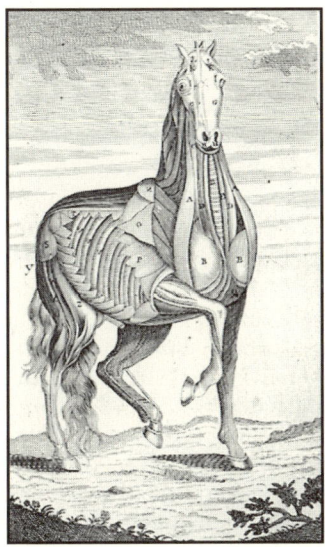

Gibson: The farrier's new guide, 1720 (603)

603.___The farrier's new guide: containing first, the anatomy of a horse...secondly, an account of all the diseases incident to horses... **1720**. London: W. Taylor. 303 pp.

A poor work compiled before the surgeon-author had turned to veterinary practice.

604.___(same) **1722**. 3rd ed, 260 pp. §

605.___A new treatise on the diseases of horses...what is necesary to the knowledge of a horse... **1751**. London: A. Millar. 464 pp.

A genuinely new work reflecting experience.

606.___(same) **1754**. 2nd ed, 2 vol, 428; 388 pp. §

607.___The true method of dieting horses. **1722**. London: W. Taylor. 236 pp.

Methods of feeding based on age and use.

608.___(same) **1726**. London: J. Osborn & T. Longman 2nd ed, 236 pp. §

609.(__) Mr. Gibson's short practical method of cure for horses: extracted from his new treatise... **1755**. London: A. Millar. 249 pp. §

A digest of the earlier work, by Gibson's son.

---

610. **GIOLO, Vincenzo.** Trattato di patologia veterinaria. **1838**. Padova: Cartallier & Sicca. 2 vol, 259; 280 pp. §

An early work on general veterinary pathology.

611. **GIRARD, Francois Narcisse** (1796-1825). A treatise on the teeth of the horse, shewing its age by the changes the teeth undergo... Trans by T.I. Ganly. **1829**. London: Sherwood, Gilbert. 75 pp.

612. **GLASS, Eugene.** The sporting bull terrier: A book of general information... **1915**. Battle Creek, MI: The Dog Fancier. 81 pp.

Characteristics; with rules for fighting.

613. **GLEASON, Oliver W.** Gleason's veterinary hand-book and system of horse taming. **1899.** Chicago: Thompson & Thomas. 520 pp. §
    A mediocre work for stock owners.
614. __(same) **1901.** 520 pp.
615. __Gleason's veterinary hand-book and system of horse training. **1900.** Chicago: G.M. Hill. 520 pp. §
    Differs only in title from item 613.
616. __Gleason's horse book and veterinary adviser comprising history...shoeing, doctoring...and general care of the horse. **1892.** Chicago: M.A. Donohue. 498 pp. §
    A comprehensive work for horsemen.
617. __Gleason's horse book: the only authorized work by America's king of horses... **1892.** Chicago: M.A. Donohue. 498 pp. §
    Identical to preceding work.
618. __How to handle and educate vicious horses: together with hints on the training and health of dogs. **1903.** New York: O. Judd. 205 pp.
    Includes a biography, shoeing and horse diseases.
619. **GOBERT, H.-J; CAGNY, P.** Le cheval de course: elevage, hygiene, entrainment, maladies. **1925.** Paris: J.-B. Bailliere. 510 pp. §
    Training, diseases and lameness of racehorses.
620. **GOEZE, Johann August Ephraim** (1731-1793). Versuch einter Naturgeschicte der Eingeweidedwurmer tierischer Korper. **1782.** Blankenburg: P.A. Pape. 471 pp.
    On helminth parasites of animals.
621. **GOODRICH, Charles Augustus** (1790-1862). A new family encyclopedia, or, compendium of universal knowledge... **1833.** Phila: [s.n.]. 4th ed, 468 pp. §
    Includes 130 pp on domestic animals & diseases.
622. **GORDON, Charles Alexander, Sir** (1821-1899). Inoculation for rabies and hydrophobia: a study of the literature on the subject. **1887.** London: Bailliere, Tindall. 127 pp. §
    A history, with doubts re: vaccine efficacy.
623. **GORHAM, Frederic P(oole)** (1871-1933). A laboratory guide for the dissection of the cat... **1899.** New York: Scribner's. 87 pp.
    A basic comparative anatomy text.
624. **GOUBAUX, Armand** (1820-1890); **BARRIER, Gustave.** The exterior of the horse. Trans by S.J.J. Harger. **1892.** Phila: J.B. Lippincott. 2nd ed, 916 pp. §
    A classic on conformation, gaits and teeth.
625. **GRAHAM, R.B. Cunninghame.** The horses of the conquest. **1930.** London: W. Heinemann. 161 pp. §
    Care of horses by 16thC conquistadores.
626. **GRAHM, Thomas C.** The cow & sheep doctor: describing the proper treatment...and medicine to be used in the cure of each distemper. **1852.** Dublin: W. Leckie. 3rd ed, 61 pp.
    Some curious treatments for curious diseases.

627. **GRAY, Ernest A(lfred)** (1908-). Man midwife: The further experiences of John Knyveton, M.D... **1946.** London: R. Hale. 210 pp. §
   Mentions Sainbel's and Hunter's connections with the London Veterinary College.
628. **GRAYBILL, Harry Webster** (1875-). Studies on the biology of the Texas-fever tick. **1911.** Washington: GPO. 42 pp. §
   Report on BAI work on Texas fever transmission.

Great Britain, Animal Disease

629.__(Abortion). Committee to inquire into epizootic abortion. **1905-13.** London: HMSO. 185 pp.
630.__Animal health: a centenary, 1865-1965. **1965.** London: HMSO. 396 pp. §
   Work of veterinary dept, Ministry of Agriculture.
631.__(Cattle trade). Report of cattle diseases prevention and cattle importation bills. **1864.** London: HMSO. 218 pp.
   Prevalence of disease in imported animals.
632.__(__). On the transatlantic cattle trade. **1891.** London: HMSO. 275 pp.
   An inquiry into care of cattle and losses at sea.
633.__(Hog cholera). Report of the departmental committee...to inquire into swine fever. **1893-97.** London: HMSO. Pt 1, 8 pp; Pt 2, 272 pp.
634.__(Louping ill). Report of the departmental committee...to inquire into...the diseases of sheep known as louping ill and braxy. **1906.** London: HMSO. 3 vol, 36; 342; 13 pp.
635.__(Pleuropneumonia). Report of the departmental committee...to inquire into pleuro-pneumonia and tuberculosis... **1888.** London: HMSO. Pt 1, 12 pp; Pt 2, 317 pp.
636.__(Rinderpest). Report...to inquire into the origin and nature of the cattle plague... **1866.** London: HMSO. 3 vol, 199; 81; 244 pp.
   Investigation of 1860 outbreak; color plates.
637.__(__). Report on the origin, propagation, nature, and treatment of the cattle plague... **1866.** London: HMSO. 59 pp.
   Statistics related to 1865 outbreak.
638.__(Statutes). Privy council office. Handbook for England, Wales and Scotland, of the laws and regulations relating to contagious and infectious diseases among animals. **1880.** London: HMSO. 445 pp.
639.__(__). New handbook... **1885.** 747 pp.
640.__(__). Handbook of the laws...[on] diseases...transit...importation of animals... **1895.** London: HMSO. 322 pp.
641.__(Tuberculosis). Report...[on] the effect of food derived from tuberculous animals on human health. **1896-1901.** London: HMSO. 23; 300 pp.
642.__(__). Report...[on] procedures for controlling danger to man through the use as food of the meat and milk of tuberculous animals. **1898.** London: HMSO. 454 pp.

643.__(__). Second interim report...[on] the relations of human and animal tuberculosis. **1907.** London: HMSO. 98 pp.
   With historical data and results of inoculation.
644.__(__). Final report... **1911-15.** London: HMSO. In 6 parts.
   Causes and lesions of TB in man and animals.

645. **GREEN, Ben K.** The village horse doctor: west of the Pecos. **1971.** New York: Knopf. 306 pp.
   Experiences of first DVM in Fort Stockton, Texas.
646. **GRENSIDE, F.C.** Essays on horse subjects. **1907.** New York: The author. 130 pp. §
   Hereditary unsoundness, shoeing, lameness, etc.
647. **GRESSWELL, Albert.** Diseases and disorders of the horse...equine medicine and surgery. **1886.** Leeds: Yorkshire Newspaper Co. 227 pp.
   By member of a noted veterinary family.
648.__; **GRESSWELL, James Brodie.** (same). **1906.** New York: W.R. Jenkins. 223 pp.
   A generally sensible work; includes anesthesia.
649. **GRESSWELL, George** (1858-1914); **GRESSWELL, Charles.** The veterinary; pharmacopoeia, materia medica, and therapeutics... **1886.** London: Bailliere, Tindall. 398 pp.
   A standard work from numerous sources.
650. **GRESSWELL, James Brodie; GRESSWELL, Albert.** The bovine prescriber...for veterinary practitioners and students. **1900.** New York: W.R. Jenkins. 2nd ed, rev by George Gresswell. 102 pp. §
   A concise pharmacopoeia.
651.__ __The equine hospital prescriber, for the use of veterinary practitioners and students. **1905.** New York: W.R. Jenkins. 3rd ed, rev by George Gresswell. 165 pp. §
652.__ __A manual of the theory and practice of equine medicine. **1885.** London: Bailliere, Tindall. 2nd ed, rev by George Gresswell. 399 pp. §
   Lacking in specific treatments.
653.__ __(same) **1890.** 2nd ed, 539 pp.
654.__ __(same) **1909.** New York: W.R. Jenkins. 2nd ed, 539 pp. §
655. **GRESSWELL, James Brodie.** Veterinary pharmacology and therapeutics. **1885.** New York: W.R. Jenkins. 206 pp.
656. **GREW, Nehemiah.** The comparative anatomy of stomachs and guts. **1681.** London: The author. 428 pp. §
   Includes horse, dog and cat, with a good description of the physiology of rumination.
657. **GRIFFITHS, William.** A practical treatise on farriery: deduced from the experience of above forty years... **1784.** Wrexham: R. Marsh. 184 pp.
   A groom's compilation of brutal treatments.

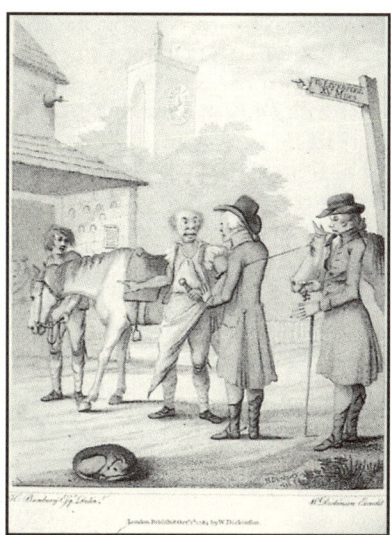

Griffiths: A practical treatise on farriery, 1795 (658)

658. __(same)...from the experience of above fifty years... **1795**. Wrexham: J. Marsh. 184 pp. §

659. **GRIMSHAW, Anne.** The horse, a bibliography of British books, 1851-1976: with a commentary on the role of the horse in British social history... **1982**. London: Library Assn; Phoenix, AZ: Oryx Press. 474 pp.

Includes many works of veterinary interest.

660. **GRISONE, Federico.** Ordini di cavalcare...et le nature de' cavalli... **1553**. Venegia: V. Valgrisi. 222 pp.

An equitation handbook by a noted riding master.

661. **GROTH, Aaron H.** Veterinary medicine: University of Missouri-Columbia, 1872-1968. **1968**? [s.l. s.n.]. 51 pp. §

History of research and teaching at Univ MO.

662. **GUENON, Francois** (1796-1855). Traite des vaches laitieres et de l'espece bovine en general. **1861**. Paris: W. Remquet. 371 pp. §

The escutcheon as indicator of milking ability.

663. **GUERRA, Francisco.** American medical bibliography 1639-1783. A chronological catalogue... **1962**. New York: L.C. Harper. 810 pp.

Includes works on veterinary medicine.

664. **GUNTHER, Friedrich August.** New manual of... homoeopathic treatment of the horse, the ox, the sheep, the dog, and other domestic animals. **1847**. Boston: O. Clapp. Trans from 3rd German ed, reprint of London ed, 408 pp.

Includes homeopathic rationale and diagnosis.

665. __(same) **1856**. 2nd American ed, 352 pp. §

666. **GUTENACKER, F.** Die Hufkrankheiten des Pferdes. **1901**? Stuttgart: F. Enke. 482 pp.

A comprehensive work on equine foot disease.

667. **HAGAN, William Arthur** (1893-1963). The infectious diseases of domestic animals... **1944.** Ithaca, NY: Comstock. 665 pp. §
   First edition of a long-since standard text.
668. **HAINES, Francis et al.** The Appaloosa horse. **1957.** Moscow: ID: News-Review Publ Co. 3rd ed, 512 pp.
669. **HALFPENNY, John.** Der englische Stall-meister und bewaerte Ross-arzt... **1765.** Leipzig: J.M.L. Teubner. 4th ed, 352 pp.
   Includes work of Matthew Hodson (item 671).

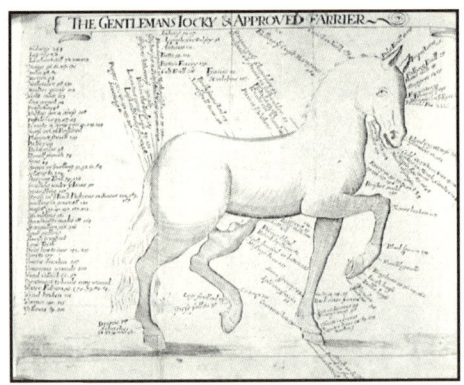

Halfpenny: The gentleman's jockey and approved farrier, 1681 (670)

670.___ The gentleman's jockey and approved farrier, instructing in the nature, causes, and cures of all diseases incident to horses... **1681.** London: H. Twyford. 6th ed, 76 pp. §
   A worthless plagiary in the manner of Markham.
671.___; **HODSON, Matthew.** (same) **1704.** London: J. Place. 9th ed, 271 pp.
   Not improved by addition of Hodson's work.
672. **HALL, Maurice Crowther** (1881-1938). Control of animal parasites: General principles and their application. **1936.** Evanston, IL: No Am Vet. 162 pp. §
   Parasite control as a military exercise.
673.___ Diagnosis and treatment of internal parasites. **1923.** Chicago: Vet Med. 102 pp. §
   An illustrated work by a noted parasitologist.
674.___(same) **1924.** 3rd ed, 92 pp. §
675.___ Worm parasites of domesticated animals: parasites of swine. **1924.** Chicago: No Am Vet. 160 pp. §
   Detailed species descriptions, lesions, treatment.
676. **HALL, R. Boylston.** Every man his own farrier: common-sense instructions for shoeing horses... **1895.** Chicago: [s.n.]. 67 pp.
   Emphasizes good foot care.
677. **HALLGREN, W.** Svensk veterinarhistoria I ord och bilder. **1960.** [s.l.]: Sveriges Veterinarforbund. 196 pp. §
   Swedish vet med from 18thC; many illustrations.

678. **HANCOCK, Reginald Cuthbert Greatrex.** Memoirs of a veterinary surgeon. **1952.** London: MacGibbon & Kee. 224 pp. §
Autobiography of an early 20thC Britisher.
679. **HANOVER, Marcus D.** A practical treatise on the law of horses, embracing the law of bargain, sale, and warranty of horses and other livestock. **1872.** Cincinnati: R. Clarke. 245 pp. §
Principles of equine jurisprudence, with cases.
680.__(same) **1875.** 2nd ed, 411 pp. §
681. **HANSON, Harry D(ennett).** Manual of prescription writing and posology: prepared for students and practitioners of veterinary medicine. **1900.** New York: [s.n.]. 230 pp.
A basic work, with extensive Latin terminology.
682.__Practice of equine medicine: a manual for students and practitioners... **1899.** New York: The author. 271 pp.
A quiz compend, with Rx for horses and dogs.
683. **HANSON, James.** Veterinary anatomy, histology, physiology and comparative anatomy. **1907.** St Joseph, MO: [s.n.]. 100 pp.
A review compend for students.
684. **HARLAN, Geo(rge) O.** Illustrated horse-owner's guide: being a synopsis of the diseases of horses and cattle... **1879.** Toledo, OH: B.F. Wade. 158 pp. §
A handbook with little useful information.
685. **HARTWIG, Adolph H.** Rural veterinary secrets...of successfully applying first aid and home remedies to ailing farm animals. **1921.** Watertown, WI: 260 pp. §
A do-it-yourself work promoting author's methods.
686. **(HARVEY, William)** (1587-1657). The works of William Harvey... Trans by Robert Willis. **1847.** London: Sydenham Society. 647 pp. §
Harvey's epochal work on circulation, embryology.
687.(__) Exercitatio anatomica de motu cordis et sanguinis in animalibus. Trans with notations by Chauncey D. Leake. **1931.** Springfield, IL: C. C Thomas. 141 pp. §
Original publication Frankfort 1628.
688. **HASELBUSH, Willard C.** Mark Morris: veterinarian. **1984.** SL: The author. 231 pp. §
Biography of a pioneer in small animal practice.
689. **HASLAM, John.** A few brief observations on the foot of the horse and on shoeing. **1832.** Baltimore: S. Harker. 14 pp. §
By an early US graduate (1803) of London school.
690. **HASSLOCH, Augustus C.** A compend of veterinary materia medica and therapeutics. **1896.** New York: W.R. Jenkins. 225 pp.
A review for students, from numerous sources.
691.__(same) **1906.** 225 pp.
692. **HAUBNER, Gottleib Karl** (1806-1882). Landwirthschaftliche Thierheilkunde...Die inneren und ausseren Krankheiten der...Haussaugethiere... **1880.** Berlin: Wiegandt, Hempel. 843 pp.
On the diseases of domestic animals for farmers.

693. **HAW, William**. Practical methods of handling horses...treatment of diseases in both horses and cattle. **1903**. Latimer, IA: S. Hanson. 112 pp.
   Gentle methods for breaking, but vile remedies.
694. **HAWKINS, B(enjamin) Waterhouse** (1807-1889). The anatomy of the horse. **1908**. London: Winsor & Newton. 148 pp. §
   Compares equine and human skeleton and muscles.
695. **HAYCOCK, William**. The gentleman's stable manual ...on construction of the stable...feeding and grooming...hygienic treatment of the sick horse... **1859**. London: Routledge, Warnes. 528 pp. §
696.__(same) **1861**. 3rd ed, 522 pp.
697.__Treatise on the principles and practice of veterinary medicine and surgery. **1858**. London: J. Churchill. 160 pp. §
   Limited to inflammation (96 pp) and wounds.
698. **HAYES, M(atthew) Horace** (1842-1904). Soundness and age of horses: a veterinary and legal guide to the examination of horses for soundness. **1887**. London: W. Thacker. 110 pp. §
   A practical manual, with detailed plates on teeth.
699.__Veterinary notes for horse owners: a manual of horse medicine and surgery... **1861**. London: W. Thacker. 4th ed, 646 pp. §
   A high-quality popular book for laymen.
700.__(same) **1897**. 5th ed, 733 pp. §
   Extensively revised; includes ageing.
701.__(same) **1915**. London: Hurst & Blackett. 833 pp. §
702.__The points of the horse: a familiar treatise on equine conformation. **1893**. London: W. Thacker. 378 pp. §
   A classic work on conformation and breeds.
703.__The points of the horse: a treatise on the conformation, movements, breeds and evolution of the horse. **1930**. London: Hurst, Blackett. 5th ed, 595 pp. §
   Illustrated by 600 photos and drawings.
704. **HAYGARTH, John** (1740-1827). A sketch of a plan to exterminate the casual small-pox from Great Britain... **1793**. London: J. Johnson. 254 pp.
   Prevalence of smallpox; plans for inoculation.
705. **HAZARD, Willis P. Ope** (1825-1913). How to select cows: or the Guenon system simplified... **1889**. Westchester, PA: The author; London: Trubner & Co. 149 pp.
   The escutcheon as indicator of milking ability.
706. **HEATLEY, George S(mith)**. The horse-owners' safeguard: a handy medical guide for every man who owns a horse. **1882**. Edinburgh: Blackwood. 232 pp.
   An unsophisticated work of doubtful utility.
707.__(same) **1895**. New York: W.R. Jenkins. 172 pp
708. **HECKER, J(ustus) F(riedrich) C(arl)** (1795-1850). The epidemics of the middle ages. Trans by B.G. Babington. **1844**. London: B. Woodfall. 418 pp. §
   A German classic, with items of vety interest.
709. **HEMENWAY, Henry Bixby** (1856-). Essentials of veterinary law. **1916**. Chicago: Am J Vet Med. 319 pp.
   Veterinary jurisprudence, with case citations.

710. **HENDERSON, R.** A treatise on the breeding of swine... **1811.** Leith: A. Allardice. 118 pp.
   Section on diseases includes other animals.
711. **(HENLEY, Walter de)** (13thC). Walter of Henley's husbandry... Trans by Elizabeth Lamond. **1890.** London; New York: Longmans, Green. 171 pp. §
   Husbandry and diseases of domestic animals.
712. **HERBERT, Henry William** (pseud Frank Forrester) (1807-1858). The complete manual for young sportsmen: with...the breaking, management, and hunting of the dog... **1857.** New York: Stringer & Townsend. 480 pp. §
   Hunting dog breeds, their management and diseases.
713. __(same) **1863.** 480 pp. §
714. __The dog. **1873.** New York: American News. 663 pp. §
   Includes Dinks: A sportsman's vade-mecum; Mayhew: Dogs and their management; Hutchinson: Dog breaking.
715. __(same) **1873.** New York: W.A. Townsend.
716. __Hints to horse-keepers...embracing how to breed a horse...how to feed...physic a horse... **1859.** New York: O. Judd. 428 pp.
   Horse care, with sections on disease and shoeing.
717. __(same) **1864.** New York: C.M. Saxton. 425 pp. §
718. __Hints to horse-keepers...embracing chapters on mules and ponies, with additions... **1887.** New York: O. Judd. 425 pp. §
719. **(HERING, Eduard von)** (1799-1881). Hering's Operationslehre fur Tierarzte. Rev by Eduard Vogel. **1885.** Stuttgart: Schickhardt & Ebner. 704 pp.
   A veterinary surgery, with many illustrations.
720. **HERPIN, Jean Charles** (1798-1872). Memoire sur une apoplexie charbonneuse de la rate... **1836.** Paris: Huzard. 23 pp.
   An outbreak of anthrax with transmission to man.
721. **HERRICK, L.R.** The horse owner's friend...diseases of horses and cattle... **1871.** New York: L. Warner. 8 pp.
   A promotion of the author's remedies.
722. **HERRLINGER, Robert** (1914-1968). History of medical illustration, from antiquity to 1600. Trans from German by Graham Fulton-Smith. **1970.** New York: Editions Medicina Rara. 178 pp. §
   With 318 illustrations, 32 plates, many in color.
723. **HERTWIG, Karl Heinrich** (1798-1881). Practisches Handbuch der Chirurgie fur Thierarzte. **1874.** Berlin: A. Hirschwald. 850 pp.
   Surgery of the horse and cow; 1st ed 1850.
724. **HERZOG, Maximilian Joseph** (1858-). A text-book on disease-producing microorganisms... **1910.** Phila; New York: Lea & Febiger. 644 pp.
   An early text on veterinary microbiology.
725. **HIBBARD, David R.** A treatise on cow-pox...small-pox...subsequent to vaccination... **1835.** New York: Harpers brothers. 69 pp.
   Reasons for occasional inefficacy of vaccination.

HIEOVER, Harry—see Charles Bindley.

726. **HILL, John Woodroffe** (-1909). The diseases of the cat. **1906**. New York: W.R. Jenkins. 123 pp. §

An insightful early work on cat diseases.

727.__The management and diseases of the dog. **1878**. New York: A. Cogswell. 383 pp.

Written "to alleviate the sufferings of the canine race," partly by eliminating spaying.

728.__(same) **1884**. New York: W.R. Jenkins. 383 pp.

729.__(same) **1890**. 383 pp. §

730.__(same) **1905**. London: S. Sonnenschein; New York: Macmillan. 531 pp.

Dosage tables and points for judging added.

John Hinds (pseud for John Badcock; fl 1816-30)

731.__Farriery taught on a new and easy plan: being a treatise on the diseases and accidents of the horse. **1852**. Phila: Lippincott, Grambo. 224 pp. §

Like Hinds: The veterinary surgeon (qv).

732.__The grooms' oracle and pocket stable directory... **1830**. London: J. Badcock. 298 pp. §

"The title alone condemns it." (Smith)

733.__The veterinary surgeon: or, farriery taught on a new and easy plan... **1830**. Phila: J. Grigg. 224 pp. §

Reprint of London 1827 ed; "An extraordinary book, full of hideous mistakes." (Smith)

734.__(same) **1833**. 224 pp. §

735.__(same) **1834**. 224 pp. §

736.__(same) **1847**. Phila: Grigg & Elliot. 224 pp. §

737.__(same) Veterinary surgery and practice of medicine, or, farriery taught on a new plan... **1829**. London: Whittaker, Treacher. 2nd ed, 581 pp.

---

739. **HINEBAUGH, Theries D.** Veterinary dental surgery, for the use of students, practitioners and stockmen. **1889**. Lafayette, IN: [s.n.]. 256 pp.

740. **HIRSCH, Fritz.** Die Todesursachen der Berliner Marstallpferde: in den jahren 1668-1887. **1935**. Berlin: Friedrich-Wilhelms Univ. 61 pp.

Causes of death in stabled horses.

741. **HOARD, William Dempster** (1836-1918). The responsibilities of the veterinarian to the dairyman: an address. **1909**. Ithaca, NY: [s.n.]. 7 pp. §

Encourages close working relationships.

742. **HOARE, E(dward) Wallis** (1863-1920). A manual of veterinary therapeutics and pharmacology. **1906**. Toronto: J.A. Carveth. 2nd ed, 779 pp.

Includes a 300 pp section on materia medica.

743.__A system of veterinary medicine. **1913-15.** Chicago: A. Eger. 2 vol, 1327; 1623 pp. §
   A multiauthor work of monumental proportions.
744. (__) Hoare's veterinary materia medica and therapeutics. Rev by J.R. Grieg and G.F. Boddie. **1942.** Chicago: A. Eger. 528 pp. §
   A first-rate update of a classic text.
745. **HOBDAY, Frederick Thomas George, Sir** (1870-1939). Fifty years a veterinary surgeon. **1938.** London: Hutchinson & Co. 288 pp. §
   By a noted educator who modernized vet surgery.
746.__Surgical diseases of the dog and cat: with chapters on anaesthetics and obstetrics. **1906.** London: Bailliere, Tindall. 2nd ed, 366 pp. §
   By a pioneer of small animal practice.
747.__(same) **1924.** Chicago: Chicago Medical Book Co. 435 pp.
748. (__) Hobday's surgical diseases of the dog and cat. Rev by J.C. McCunn. **1953.** Baltimore: Williams & Wilkins. 6th ed, 453 pp.
   An updated version of a long-standard work.
749. **HODGINS, Joseph Edmund** (1872-); **HASKETT, Thomas Henry** (1873-). The veterinary science: the anatomy, diseases and treatment of domestic animals... **1897.** Detroit: Veterinary Science Co. 13th ed, 416 pp. §
   A mediocre work for farmers.
750.__(same) **1905.** 56th ed, 416 pp.
751. **HOGE, Moses Drury** (1861-1920). Diagnostic urinalysis. **1910.** Richmond, VA: Dietz Printing. 93 pp.
   On renal function and urinalysis.
752. **HOGG, Jabez** (1817-1899). The microscope: its history, construction, and applications... **1856.** London: H. Ingram. 2nd ed, 457 pp. §
   A comprehensive work with many illustrations.
753.__(same) **1861.** 5th ed, 621 pp. §
754. (**HOHMAN, John George**). John George Hohman's pow-wows, or, long lost friend: a collection of...remedies for man as well as animals. **1819?** [s.l. s.n.]. 94 pp.
   A Penna-German "hex book" containing charms and magic against animal and human ailments.
755. **HOLMES, S.J.** The evolution of animal intelligence. **1911.** New York: Henry Holt. 296 pp. §
   From evolution of instinct to simian mentality.
756. (**HOMEOPATHY**). A manual of homoeopathic veterinary practice: designed for horses, all kinds of domestic animals and fowls... **1874.** New York; Phila: Boericke & Tafel. 684 pp. §
   Includes rationale of treatment; surgery.
757.__(same) **1874.** Phila: F.E. Boericke. 2nd ed, 684 pp. §
758.__(same) **1879.** New York; Phila: Boericke & Tafel. 2nd ed, 684 pp. §
759.__Manuel de medecine veterinaire homoeopathique: indiquant le traitement des maladies de tous les animaux domestiques... **1837.** Paris: Bailliere. 299 pp.
   From German work; for veterinarians and owners.

HOPE, Sir William—see Jacques Solleysel

760. **HOPKINS, Grant Sherman** (1865-). Guide to the dissection and study of the blood vessels and nerves of the limbs, thorax and abdomen of the horse. **1925.** Ithaca, NY: NY State Vet College. 53 pp + plates. §

A detailed guide with excellent plates.

761.__Guide to the dissection and study of the cranial nerves and blood vessels of the horse. **1922.** [s.l. s.n.]. 41 pp + plates. §

762. **HORNIDY, O. Evans.** A treatise on hog cholera and chicken cholera...their cure and prevention. **1879.** Davenport, IA: Egbert, Fidlar. 91 pp.

Speculation on cause, with "certain" remedies.

Horse

763.__Anatomical model of the mare. **1900?** New York: Amer Thermo-ware Co. 5 pp. §

Five color plates with fold-out body parts.

764.__The Arabian horse bibliography: a project of the Arabian Horse Trust with...annotations by Ruth E. Boyd... **1985.** Westminster: The Trust. 180 pp.

Includes many 18th-19thC works (Youatt, Gibson, Beringer, etc, with sections on diseases).

765.__The horse, its varieties and management in health and disease. **1870?** London: F. Warne. 259 pp.

A generally sensible work for owners.

766.__How to buy a horse: containing instructions for...first treatment of some injuries and diseases... **1840.** London: Sherwood, Gilbert. 250 pp.

On defects and diseases in relation to purchase.

767.__Indian horse notes...for ready reference on emergencies specially adapted for officers... **1906.** Calcutta: Thacker, Spink. 6th ed, 101 pp.

Mainly first aid; includes Hindustani vocabulary.

768.__The horseman's handbook: a compendium of useful information for every horse owner. **1904.** Chicago: Magnus Flaws & Co. 146 pp. §

Deals mainly with trotting horses.

769.__Pennetegninger af dyrlaege Sander-Larsen. **1886.** Horsens, Denmark: Elisedal. 26 plates.

An atlas of equine anatomy.

770.__Oft probirtes und bewahrt erfundenes Ross-arznei-buchlein... **1700?** Augsburg: [s.n.]. 56 pp.

A brief work on equine disease.

771.__Pratts pointers on the horse, including breeding...stabling, diseases, etc... **1892.** Phila: Pratt Food Co. 176 pp.

A promotion of Pratt's remedies

772.__(same) **1898.** 176 pp. §

773.__(same) **1905.** 183 pp. §

774.__Simplicissimus, der Deutsche Pferdearzt, oder, eine kritische Zusammenstellung der... Pferdekrankheiten. **1847**. [s.l. s.n.]. 92 pp. §
  On treatment of equine diseases.

775. **HOUCK, Ulysses Grant** (1866-1934). The Bureau of Animal Industry...its establishment, achievements and current activities. **1924**. Washington: The author. 390 pp. §
  The epochal work of the BAI from 1884 to 1920.
776. **HOUDETOT, Cesar Francois Adolphe** (1799-1869). La petite venerie, ou, la chasse au chien courant. **1855**. Paris: Depot de Librairie. 352 pp. §
  A work on hunting dogs.
777. **HOWARD, Robert W.** The horse in America. **1965**. Chicago: Follett. 298 pp. §
  Origin and development, with many historic photos.
778. **HOWDEN, Peter.** Horse warranty. A plain and comprehensive guide to the various points to be noted... **1862**. London: R. Hardwicke. 160 pp. §
  On soundness and legal aspects of warranty. Second copy with S.B. Nelson signature.
779. **HOWE, A.H.** The horseman's pocket companion: a new system of horse training. **1870**. Newark, NJ: Newark Courier. 30 pp.
780. **HOWE, Murray.** Stable conversation. **1900**. Chicago: Horse Review Co. 262 pp. §
  A satire on race track characters.
781. **HOWEY, M. Oldfield.** The horse in magic and myth. **1923**. London: Rider. 238 pp. §
  Early beliefs about horses; chapter on centaurs.
782. **HOWEY, W. Oldfield.** The cat in the mysteries of religion and magic. **1955**. New York: A. Richmond. 254 pp. §
  Feline symbolism and myths through the ages.
783. **HUBBARD, Clifford L.B.** An introduction to the literature of British dogs: five centuries of illustrated dog books. **1949**. Ponterwyd, Wales: [s.n.]. 56 pp. §
  Works of Caius, Turberville, Markham, etc.
784. **HUIDEKOPER, Rush Shippen** (1854-1901). Age of the domestic animals. Being a complete treatise on the dentition of the horse, ox, sheep, hog, and dog... **1891**. Phila; London: F.A. Davis. 217 pp. §
  Tooth structure and eruption; detailed plates.
785. (**HUISH, C.H.**). The causes of and remedy for sterility in mares, cows, sheep & bitches... **1910**. London: C.H. Huish. 112 pp. §
  Promotes use of artificial insemination.
786. **HUMPHREYS, F(rederick)** (1816-1900). Manual of veterinary specific homeopathy, comprising diseases of horses, cattle, sheep, hogs, and dogs... **1860**. New York: J.A. Gray. 240 pp.
  Treatment based on secret remedies; barn chart.
787.__(same) **1886**. New York: Humphreys' Homeopathic Co. 4th ed, 416 pp.
788.__(same) **1901**. 5th ed, 433 pp. §

789. **HUNTING, William** (18846-1913). The art of horse-shoeing: A manual for farriers. **1898.** New York: W.R. Jenkins. 129 pp.

A practical work by a noted veterinarian.

790.__(same) **1922.** London: Bailliere, Tindall. 4th ed, rev by A.B. Mattinson. 220 pp. §

791. **(HUSBANDRY).** The complete grazier: or, gentleman's and farmer's directory. 1776. London: J. Almon. 252 pp.

Husbandry and diseases of domestic animals.

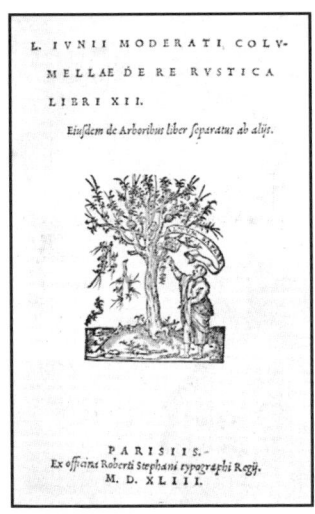

Libri de re rustica, 1543 (792)

792.__Libri de rustica: M. Catonis...Varronis... **1543.** Paris: Roberti Stephani. 2 vol, 186; 312 pp. §

Roman husbandry, with sections on animal disease.

793.__Scriptores rei rusticae veteres latini: Cato, Varro, Columella, Palladius...Vegetius... **1781.** Mannhemii: Cura...Societatis Literatae. §

Includes Vegetius: Books of the veterinary art.

794. **HUTYRA, Ferenc** (1860-1934); **MAREK, Joseph** (1868-). Special pathology and therapeutics of domestic animals. Trans by J.R Mohler and A. Eichhorn. **1913.** Chicago: A. Eger. 2 vol, 1st American from 3rd German ed. 1113; 1018 pp. §

Includes brief history of each disease.

795.__(same) **1916-17.** 2nd American from 4th German ed, 2 vol, 1213; 1108 pp. §

796. **HYDE, James Nevine** (1840-1910). A practical treatise on diseases of the skin... **1901.** Phila; New York: Lea Bros. 6th ed, 828 pp.

For medical students and physicians.

797. **JACKSON, Oscar C.** Dr. Oscar C. Jackson's veterinary medicines... **1887.** Jamaica, NY: Long Island Farmer. 113 pp. §
 Homeopathic treatment based on secret remedies.
798. **JACQUES, Daniel Harrison** (1825-1877). New illustrated rural manuals: comprising the house, the farm, the garden, domestic animals... **1859.** New York: Fowler & Wells. 646 pp. §
 Section on animals (168 pp) includes diseases.
799. **JAKOB, Heinrich** (1874-). Diagnose und Therapie der inneren Krankheiten des Hundes. **1913.** Stuttgart: F. Enke. 636 pp.
 An early text on canine medicine.
800. **JAMES, Robert Kent** (ed). The Angora cat...history, peculiarities and diseases... **1898.** Boston: James Bros. 102 pp. §
 On care, breeding, training and disease.
801. **JARDINE, William, Sir** (1800-1874). The naturalist's library...Mammalia... **1833.** Edinburgh: W.H. Lizars. 267 pp. §
 Zoology of the canine genus, with 31 color plates.
802. **JARVIS, D.C.** Folk medicine: A Vermont doctor's guide to good health. **1958.** New York: Henry Holt. 182 pp. §
 Touts vinegar for human and animal diseases.
803. **JASPER, D(onald) E(dward)** (1918-). A short history of the School of Veterinary Medicine, University of California. **1964.** Davis, CA: Simmons. 49 pp. §
 Signed by author.
804. **JEFFERIS, Benjamin Grant** (1851-). The household guide, or, domestic encyclopedia: home remedies for man and beast... **1895.** Naperville, IL: J.L. Nichols. 521 pp. §
 With 85 pp on breaking horses and animal disease.
805. **JENNINGS, Robert** (1924-1893). Cattle and their diseases: embracing their history and breeds...the diseases to which they are subject, and the remedies best adapted to their cure. **1890.** Phila: Keystone Publishing Co. 340 pp. §
 Book for farmers, by first secretary of USVMA.
806.__The horse and his diseases...[with] the remedies best adapted to their cure. **1860.** Phila: Keystone Publ. 390 pp. §
 For owners; includes Rarey's horse taming.
807.__(same) **1863.** Phila: J.E. Potter. 384 pp. §
808.__Horse-training made easy: being a new and practical system of...educating the horse... **1866.** Phila: J.E. Potter. 186 pp. §
 Promotes his remedies for equine diseases.
809. **JEWETT, Paul.** The New-England farrier, or, a compendium of farriery...wherein most of the diseases to which horses, neat cattle, sheep and swine are incident, are treated of... **1821.** Exeter, NH: John J. Williams. 54 pp. §
 Perhaps the first (1st ed 1795) work native to US.

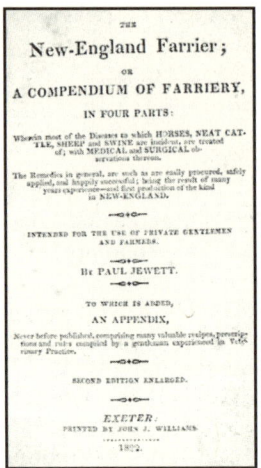

Jewett: 1822 (810)

810.__(same) **1822**. 2nd ed, 105 pp. §
811.__(same) **1826**. Exeter, NH: Josiah Richardson. New ed, 112 pp, 24 plates.
812.__The New England farrier, or, farmer's receipt book...for the cure of diseases in horses, cattle, sheep & swine... **1835**. Boston: C. Gaylord. 214 pp.
813.(__) The New-England farrier, and family physician: containing...Paul Jewett's farriery...a collection of brutal receipts...receipts for human diseases... **1828**. Exeter: Josiah Richardson. 492 pp. §

A compilation of animal and human remedies.

814. **JODELLE, Etienne** (1532-1573). Ode de la chasse. **1872**. Paris: A Lemerre. 28 pp. §

Reprint of a 16thC work on hunting.

815. **JOHNSON, C.** The farmer's encyclopedia and dictionary of rural affairs... **1844**. Phila: Carey & Hart. 1165 pp. §

Includes entries relating to domestic animals.

816. **JOHNSON, J.W.** Homoeopathic veterinary hand-book, for the farmer, stockman and horse owner. Giving...symptoms and remedies for all diseases of the horse, ox, sheep, swine and dog. **1879**. Cleveland: Ohio Farmer. 128 pp. §

Of doubtful utility, but gives specific dosages.

817. **JOHNSON, Thomas Burgeland** (1840-). The hunting directory: containing...the method of feeding and managing...hounds...their diseases, with a certain cure for distemper... **1830**. London: Sherwood, Gilbert. 312 pp. §

Extensive discussion of distemper and rabies.

818. **JOHNSTONE, James Hope Stewart** (1861-). The horse book: practical treatise on the American horse breeding industry... **1912**. Chicago: Breeder's Gazette. 271 pp. §

Breeds and breeding of farm horses.

819. **JUHANNA IBN SARAPION** (fl 9thC). Serapionis medici arabis celeberrimi practica...studiosis medicinae... **1550**. Venetiis: Apud Iuntas. 200 pp.
   A work on early Arabic medicine.
820. **JULIENNE, Pierre** (1906-). La tuberculose bovine: comment s'en debarrasser. **1938**. Paris: Flammarion. 82 pp. §
   On causes and control of bovine tuberculosis.
821. **KARASSZON, Denes.** A concise history of veterinary medicine. **1988**. Budapest: Akademiai Kiado. 458 pp.
   A first-class work, including cultural aspects.
822. **KATCHER, Aaron H.; BECK, Alan M.** (eds). New perspectives on our lives with companion animals. **1983**. Phila: Univ Penn Press. 588 pp. §
   Societal role of animals; pet-facilitated therapy
823. **KATIC, Ivan.** Dansk-russike veterinaere forbindelser 1796-1976. **1982**. Kobenhaven: [s.n.]. 317 pp. §
   A history of Danish-Russian veterinary relations.
824. __World atlas of veterinary emblems. **1987**. Copenhagen: [s.n.]. 119 pp. §
   Depicts ca 400 emblems, logos, from 48 countries.
825. __(same) **1991**. Copenhagen: Veterinaerhistorisk Forskning. 2nd ed, 150 pp. §
   Depicts ca 600 emblems, logos, from 55 countries. Inscribed by compiler to J.F. Smithcors.
826. **KAUPP, Benjamin Franklyn** (1874-). Animal parasites and parasitic diseases. **1908**. Chicago: A. Eger. 207 pp. §
   An illustrated taxonomic work.
827. __(same) **1910**. 2nd ed, 211 pp.
828. __(same) **1914**. 3rd ed, 238 pp. §
829. __Poultry diseases, with a chapter on the anatomy of the fowl. **1917**. Chicago: Am Vet Publ Co. 2nd ed, 245 pp. §
   An early work on poultry diseases and parasites.
830. **KEITH, Thomas B.** The horse interlude: a pictorial history of horse and man in the inland Northwest. **1976**. Moscow, ID: Univ Idaho Press. 195 pp.
831. **KENDALL, B(urney) J(ames)** (1845-). The doctor at home...treating the diseases of man and the horse. **1887**. Enosburg, VT: The author. 96 pp. §
   A mediocre work promoting the author's remedies.
832. __A treatise on the horse and his diseases... the symptoms, cause, and the best treatment of each. **1880**. Chicago: Rand, McNally. 91 pp. §
   Essentially the same as preceding item.
833. __(same) **1881**. Enosburg Falls, VT: The author. 95 pp. §
834. __(same) **1884**. Chicago: Rand, McNally. 91 pp. §
835. __A treatise on the horse and his diseases...covering the common ailments of horses... **1942**. Enosburg Falls, VT: The author. 80 pp. §
   Little changed from previous editions.
836. **KESTER, Wayne O.** The history of the American Association of Equine Practitioners, 1954-1979. **1980**. Golden, CO: AAEP. 160 pp. §
   A year-by-year account, by AAEP Exec Secy.

837. **KIMBALL, Victor Gage.** Veterinary state board questions and answers. **1914.** Phila; London: J.B. Lippincott. 465 pp.
  A revealing look at early state boards.
838.__(same) **1917.** 2nd ed, 395 pp. §
839.__(same) **1920.** 3rd ed, 365 pp. §
840. **KINSLEY, Albert Thomas** (1877-1941). Swine diseases. **1914.** Kansas City: Am Vet Supply Co. 238 pp.
  On diseases and treatment, with color plates.
841.__A text book of veterinary pathology, for students and practitioners. **1910.** Chicago: A. Eger. 400 pp. §
  An early text on the subject; J.V. Lacroix copy.
842.__(same) **1915.** 2nd ed, 404 pp.
843. **KIRBY, F.O.** Veterinary medicine and surgery in diseases and injuries of the horse. **1883.** New York: W. Wood. 332 pp. §
844. **KIRK, Hamilton.** Canine distemper, its complications, sequelae, and treatment. **1922.** London: Bailliere, Tindall. 236 pp. §
  The first comprehensive work on canine distemper.
845.__The diseases of the cat and its general management. **1925.** Chicago: A. Eger. 418 pp.
  An early work on feline disease, by noted DVM.
846.__Index of diagnosis (clinical and radiological) for the canine and feline surgeon, with treatment. **1939.** Baltimore: Williams & Wilkins. 561 pp.
  A different approach; E.A. Ehmer signature.
847. **KIRKEMINDE, Patricia B(arclay)** (1924-). History of veterinary medicine in Tennessee. **1976.** Nashville: Modern Typographers. 450 pp. §
  Mostly 20thC, with many anecdotes, biographies.
848. (**KIRKES, Willian Senhouse**) (1823-1864). Kirkes' handbook of physiology. Rev by C.W. Greene. **1913.** New York: W. Wood. 761 pp.
  A basic human text; E.A. Ehmer signature.
849. **KITT, Theodor** (1858-1941). Der Tierarztliche beruf und seine Geschicte. **1932.** Stuttgart: F. Enke. 63 pp. §
  History of the German veterinary profession.
850.__Atlas der Thierkrankheiten; 40 Figuren in Farbendruck uber pathologisch-anatomische Praparate... **1896.** Stuttgart: F. Enke.
  A remarkable depiction of lesions in color.
851.__Textbook of comparative general pathology, for practitioners and students of veterinary medicine. Trans by W.W. Cadbury. **1906.** Chicago: W.T. Keener. 471 pp. §
  A classic work; 2nd copy, E.E. Wegner signature.
852. **KLIMMER, Martin** (1873-). Veterinarhygiene. Grundriss der Gesundheitspflege der...Haustiere. **1908.** Berlin: P. Parey. 439 pp.
  Feeding, management and diseases of livestock.
853.__Veterinary hygiene, care of health and...contagious diseases of domesticated animals. Trans by A.A. Leibold. **1923.** Chicago: A. Eger. 431 pp. §
  An early text on preventive veterinary medicine.

854. **KNOWLSON, John C.** The Yorkshire cattle-doctor & farrier...written in plain language, which those who can read may easily understand. **1834.** London: Simpkin, Marshall. Rev ed, 272 pp.
    A mediocre work based on 72 years of experience!

855. **KOBERT, Rudolf** (1854-1918). Practical toxicology for physicians and students. Trans by L.H. Friedburg. **1897.** New York: W.R. Jenkins. 201 pp.
    Text used at American Vet Coll; E.E. Wegner copy.

856. **KOCH, Robert** (1843-1910). Aetiology of tuberculosis. Trans by T. Saure. Transactions of Massachusetts VMA. **1890.** New York: W.R. Jenkins. 97 pp.
    Results of Koch's epochal investigations.

857. **KOGER, L(avon) M.** 1899-1974 diamond jubilee, College of Veterinary Medicine, Washington State University. **1974.** Pullman, WA: Pullman Printers. Unpaged. §
    Includes roster of faculty and graduates.

858. **KOOGLE, J.D.** The farmer's own book: a treatise on the numerous diseases of the horse... **1857.** Baltimore: McCoull & Slater. 226 pp. §
    Of doubtful utility, with many domestic receipts.

859. __(same)...also a treatise on the diseases of horned cattle. **1858.** Middletown, MD: Author. 261 pp. §

860. **KORINEK, Charles James** (1880-). Diseases of domestic animals and poultry: their cause, symptoms and treatment. **1915.** Portland, OR: Author. 192 pp. §
    For farmers; promotes the author's remedies.

861. __The veterinarian. **1916.** Joliet, IL; Toronto: Gerlach-Barklow. 2nd ed, 256 pp. §
    A mediocre work for farmers.

862. **LA TOUR, Gaetan de.** Guide pratique du chasseur: contenant...le dressage des chevaux et des chiens...traitement de leurs maladies... **1876?** Paris: Laplace, Sanchez. 356 pp. §
    On hunting, including diseases of hunting dogs.

863. **LACROIX, John Victor** (1882-). Animal castration. **1915.** Chicago: Am J Vet Med. 144 pp. §
    Castration and spaying of animals and poultry.

864. __Lameness of the horse. **1916.** Chicago: Am J Vet Med. 261 pp. §
    A classic work by a noted veterinarian.

865. __(ed). Canine—Feline practice. **1936.** Evanston, IL: No Am Vet. 63 pp. §
    Extracts from North American Veterinarian.

866. __; **HOSKINS, H. Preston** (eds). Canine Surgery. **1939.** Evanston, IL: No Am Vet. 148 pp. §
    Forerunner of standard text on the subject.

867. __; **KHUEN, E.C.** (eds). Veterinary therapeutics: notes and abstracts. **1935.** Evanston, IL: No Am Vet. 64 pp. §
    Extracts from North American Veterinarian.

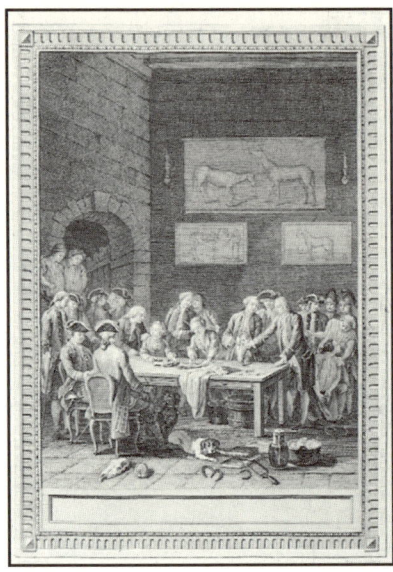

Lafosse: Cours d'hippiatrique, 1772 (868)

868. **LAFOSSE, Philippe-Etienne** (1738?-1820). Cours d'hippiatrique, ou traite complet de la medecine des chevaux... **1772.** Paris: College de Presle. 402 pp.

A monumental work on equine anatomy and disease, with 65 magnificent large folio plates.

869. ___Guide du marechal: ouvrage contenant une connoissance exacte du cheval...de guerir ses maladies... **1768.** Paris: Desaint. 426 pp. §

Management and diseases of horses, with an enlightened system of shoeing; many plates.

870. **LAFOSSE, Etienne-Guillaume** (-1765). Observations and discoveries made upon horses: with a new method of shoeing. **1755.** London: J. Nourse. 120 pp. §

A highly original work by the father of P-E. Lafosse, translated from the French.

871. **LA RUE, Adolphe de; CHERVELLE, M.; BELLECROIX, E.** Le chiens d'arret: Francois et Anglais. **1886.** Paris: Librairie de Firmin-Didot. 3rd ed, 281 pp.

Breeds of French and English hunting dogs.

872. **LAMB, Cornelius.** The western farrier: in which the principal diseases of horses are described... **1841.** Terre Haute, IN: G.A. Chapman. 160 pp.

A retrograde work with many brutal remedies.

873. **LANDER, G(eorge) D(ruce).** Veterinary toxicology. **1912.** Chicago: A. Eger. 312 pp. §

A British work with much on poisonous plants.

874. **LARIEUX, E.; JUMAUD, P.** Le chat: races, elevage, maladies. 1926. Paris: Vigot Freres. 272 pp. §

Includes breeds, history, anatomy and diseases.

James Law (1838-1921)

875.___The farmer's veterinary advisor. A guide to the prevention and treatment of disease in domestic animals. **1876.** Ithaca, NY: The author. 426 pp. §

876.___(same) **1880.** 4th ed. 426 pp.

877.___(same) **1900.** 12th ed, 617 pp, §

878.___The horseman's friend and veterinary advisor: a complete and handy treatise on domestic animals... **1907.** London: A. Moring. 439 pp. §
   Like item 875, with added material on horses.

879.___The lung plague of cattle: contagious pleuro-pneumonia. **1880.** Ithaca, NY: The author. 97 pp. §
   The nature of the disease, with extensive history.

880.___Text book of veterinary medicine, Vol 1. **1896.** Ithaca, NY: The author. 411 pp. §
   Diagnosis, fever, catarrh, roaring, heaves, etc.

881.___(same) Vol 2, **1900.** 574 pp. §
   Enteritis ,colic, bloat, azoturia, poisons, etc.

882.___(same) Vol 3, **1901.** 601 pp. §
   Nervous system, eye, milk fever, osteoporosis, etc.

883.___(same) Vol 4, **1902.** 675 pp.
   Dourine, glanders, rabies, anthrax, tetanus, etc.

884.___(same) Vol 5. **1903.** 532 pp.
   Parasites, actinomycosis, snake bite, etc.

885.___(same) **1905-06.** 2nd ed, vol 1-4; 566; 595; 611; 718 pp. §

886.___(same) **1912.** 3rd ed, Vol 4 (only), 787 pp. §

887.___Tuberculosis in cattle, and its control. **1898.** Ithaca, NY: Cornell AES Bulletin 150. 30 pp. §

---

888. **LAWRENCE, John** (1753-1839). A general treatise on cattle, the ox, the sheep, and the swine...their breeding, management, improvement and diseases. **1805.** London: H.D. Symonds. 639 pp. §
   An advocate of enlightened veterinary practice.

889.___(same) **1809.** London: Sherwood, Neely. 2nd ed, 618 pp.

890.___The history and delineation of the horse, in all his varieties...with a particular investigation of the race-horse... **1809.** London: J. Cundee. 288 pp.
   Good on management; urges humane methods.

891.___The horse in all his varieties and uses: his breeding, rearing and managment ...preservation from disease. **1829.** London: M. Arnold. 315 pp. §
   Largely abstracted from his other works.

892.___(same) **1830.** Phila: E.L. Carey & A. Hart. 238 pp. §

893.___The new farmer's calendar: or, monthly remembrancer...with the management of livestock. **1802.** London: H.D. Symonds. 4th ed, 554 pp.

894.___A philosophical and practical treatise on horses, and on the moral duties of man towards the brute creation. **1796.** London: T. Longman. 2 vol, 600; 391 pp.
   A discursive work; includes earlier writers.

895.__(same) **1802**. London: H.D. Symonds. 2nd ed, 2 vol, 639; 391 pp. §

896. **LAWRENCE, Richard.** The complete farrier and British sportsman: containing...the structure and animal economy of the horse...prevention and cure for every disease... **1816**. London: W. Lewis. 512 pp.

An ordinary compilation, except for his original naked-eye analysis of the gallop.

897.__(same) **1833**. London: T. Kelly. 518 pp. §

898.__(same) **1850**. 518 pp.

899.__An inquiry into the structure and animal economy of the horse: comprehending the diseases to which his limbs and feet are subject...shoeing, and...ascertaining his age... **1801**. Birmingham: Knott & Lloyd. 221 pp, 33 plates. §

Good on conformation and gait; exquisite plates.

900.__(same) **1803?** 2nd ed, 224 pp.

901. **LAWSON, A.** The modern farrier, or, the art of preserving the health and curing the diseases of horses, dogs, oxen, sheep, and swine. **1822**. Newcastle upon Tyne: MacKenzie & Dent. 616 pp.

An ordinary but immensely popular work.

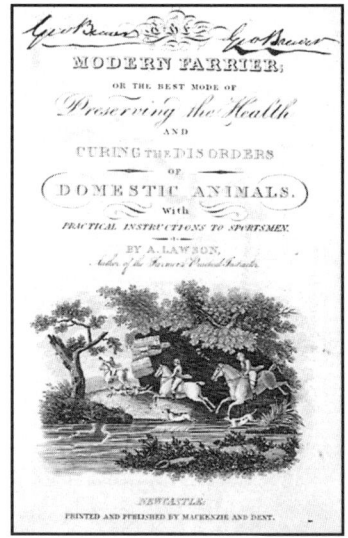

Lawson: 1825 (902)

902.__(same) **1825**. London: G. Virtue. 616 pp.

903.__(same) **1826**. London: MacKenzie & Dent. 9th ed, 616 pp.

904.__(same) **1832**. 16th ed, 616 pp.

905.__(same) **1838**. London: G. Virtue. 22nd ed, 616 pp.

906.__(same) **1846**. 28th ed, 616 pp. §

907. **LAWSON, Stephen.** An essay on the use of mixed and compressed cattle fodder...on ship-board, in camps, or in garrisons... **1797**. London: The author. 88 pp.

Promotes use of author's product.

908. **LECLAINCHE, Emanuel** (1861-1953). Histoire de la medecine veterinaire. **1936.** Toulouse: Office du Livre. 812 pp. §

A classic work,from antiquity to 20thC, with details on veterinary schools worldwide; J.V. Lacroix copy; 2nd copy L.A. Merillat signature.

909.(__) Histoire illustree de la medecine veterinaire. **1955.** Monaco: Editions Albin Michel. Foreword by Gaston Ramon. 2 vol, 249; 247 pp. §

Lavishly illustrated; text based on classic work.

910. **LECLERC, Daniel** (1652-1728). A natural and medicinal history of worms bred in the bodies of men and other animals...and the remedies which destroy them... **1721.** London: J. Wilcox. 436 pp.

Includes worms of dogs, cats and cattle.

911. **LEFEBVRE des NOETTES, Richard** (1856-). L'attelage: Le cheval de selle a travers les ages... **1931.** Paris: A. Picard. 312 pp. §

Horses and equitation throughout the ages.

912. **LEHMAN, Henry Harvey** (1868-). Lehman's poultry doctor. A treatise on poultry diseases... **1909.** Ashland, OH: The author. 96 pp. §

An early work on the subject, for farmers.

913. **LEHMANN, Karl Gotthelf** (1812-1863). Precis de chimie physiologique animale. **1855.** Paris: V. Masson. 395 pp. §

Physiological chemistry, including tissue studies.

914. **LEIB, Isaac.** Wohlerfahrner Pferde-arzt: enhaltend...Krankheiten...der Pferde... **1842.** Lebanon, PA: J. Hartman. 184 pp.

A Pennsylvania-German work on equine diseases.

915.__(same) **1860.** Lebanon: H.H. Roedel. 184 pp.

916. **LEMONDS, Leo L.** (1923-). A century of veterinary medicine in Nebraska. **1982.** Hastings, NE: The author. 395 pp. §

Includes biographies and roster of veterinarians; copiously illustrated; author's signature.

917. **LEONARD, Ellis P(ierson).** A Cornell heritage: veterinary medicine, 1868-1908. **1979.** Ithaca, NY: NYS Coll Vet Med. 288 pp. §

The early years, with accounts of first faculty.

918.__In the James Law tradition, 1908-1948. **1982.** Ithaca, NY: NYS Coll Vet Med. 342 pp.

The later years, with emphasis on the faculty.

919.__A veterinary centennial in New York State, 1890-1990. Ed by J.L. Leonard. **1989.** Ithaca, NY: NYS Vet Med Soc. 388 pp.

An account of organized vet med in New York.

920. **LEONARD, John Lynn.** First aid to animals. **1924.** New York; London: Harper. 346 pp.

921. **LESURE, J.G.** Dr. Lesure's warranted veterinary remedies... **1908.** Harrisburg, PA: The author. 128 pp. §

---

922. **LIAUTARD, Alexandre Francois Augustin** (1835-1918). Animal castration. **1884.** New York: W.R. Jenkins; London: Bailliere, Tindall. 148 pp. §

Castration and spaying of domestic species.

923.__(same) **1889**. New York: W.R. Jenkins. 4th ed, 165 pp.
924.__(same) **1902**. 12th ed. 165 pp. §
925.__(same) **1904**. 165 pp.
926.__How to tell the age of the domestic animals. **1892**. New York: W.R. Jenkins. 35 pp. §
   With 8-p Jenkins veterinary book catalog.
927.__(same) **1910**. 33 pp. §
928.__Lameness of horses and diseases of the locomotory apparatus. **1890**. New York: W.R. Jenkins. 2nd ed, 313 pp.
   Includes extracts from European writers.
929.__A manual of operative veterinary surgery. **1891**. New York: W.R. Jenkins. 786 pp. §
   General and special surgery; many illustrations.
930.__(same) **1892**. 786 pp. §
   Inscribed by author to Professor McFadyean.
931.__(same) **1906**. 803 pp. §
932.__Vade mecum of equine anatomy: for the use of advanced students and veterinary surgeons. **1879**. New York: Amer Vet Coll. 197 pp. §
   Author was dean of American Veterinary College.

---

933. **LIEBIG, Justus von** (1803-1873). Principles of agricultural chemistry. **1855**. London: Walton & Maberly. 136 pp.
   A brief work for farmers.
934.__The natural laws of husbandry. Ed by John Blyth. **1863**. New York: D. Appleton. 387 pp. §
   A classic work on agricultural chemistry.
935. **LIEGEOIS, F.** Precis de droit veterinaire...la medecine legale veterinaire...la legislation professionelle. **1934**. Paris: Librairie Agricole. 224 pp. §
   Includes warranty, contracts, rights, obligations.
936. **LINDLEY, W(illiam) H.** A history of veterinary medicine in Mississippi to 1972. **1972**. Raymond, MS: Mississippi VMA. 224 pp. §
   Mainly 20thC; many photos, list of members.
937. **LINDSAY, W(illiam) Lauder** (1829-1880). Mind in the lower animals in health and disease. **1879**. London: C.K. Paul. 2 vol, 543; 571 pp. §
   An early work on animal psychology, educability.
938. **LINTON, Robert George** (1882-). Animal nutrition and veterinary dietetics. **1927**. New York: W. Wood. 399 pp. §
   On feedstuffs and rations; J.V. Lacroix signature.
939. (**LISTER, Joseph**) (1827-1912). Lister and the ligature. **1925**. [s.l.]: Johnson & Johnson. 89 pp.
   Extracts from Lister's writings.
940. (**LIVESTOCK**). Illustrated American horse book: containing a plain, practical and improved treatment... **1878**. Chicago: Live-Stock Publ Co. 286 pp. §
   Includes The American cattle book, pp 347-390; The American swine book, pp 437-471; The American sheep book, pp 514-558.

941.__(same) **1880**. [?]
  Like 1878 ed, but with homeopathic dept added.
942.__Illustrated American Stock Book...the horse, cattle, swine, sheep & poultry... **1889**. Chicago: American Live Stock Publ Co. 615 pp. §
  A mediocre work with numerous harsh remedies.
943.__(same) **1890**. 615 pp. §
944.__(same) **1893**. 615 pp.
945.__International illustrated stock book. **1900**? Minneapolis: International Stock Food Co. 160 pp. §
  A promotion of stock feeds and remedies.
946.__Prose and poetry of the live stock industry of the United States. With outlines of the origin and ancient history of our live stock animals... **1959**. New York: Antiquarian Press. 757 pp.
  Many early illustrations; some disease references.
947. **LIVINGSTON, Robert R.** (1746-1813). Essays on sheep: their varieties—account of the Merinoes of Spain, France, etc. **1810**. Concord, NH: D. Cooledge. 164 pp. §
  Book hastened introduction of Merinoes into US.
948.__(same) **1813**. 143 pp. §
949. **LLORENTE LAZARO, Ramon.** Compendio de la veterinaria espanola... **1856**. Madrid: Angel Calleja. 204 pp.
  Describes works of 16th-19thC Spanish authors.
950. **LOEW, Franklin M.** (1939-); **WOOD, Edward H.**(1949-) Vet in the saddle: John L. Poett, first veterinary surgeon of the North West Mounted Police. **1978**. Saskatoon: Western Producer Prairie Books. 128 pp. §
  Life on the Canadian frontier in the late 1800s.
951. **LORD, William C.** Gastritis mucosa, or, the present epidemic among horses, commonly called influenza... **1865**. London: Longman, Green. 58 pp. §
  Signs, cause and prevention of "distemper."
952. **LOVEJOY, Andrew James** (1845-). Forty years' experience of a practical hog man... **1914**. Springfield, IL. 170 pp. §
  On swine breeding and management.
953. **LUCAS, A.T.** Furze: A survey and history of its uses in Ireland. **1960**. Dublin: Natl Museum. 203 pp. §
  References to animal fodder and cures.
954. **LUDLOW, Jacob R(apelye)** (1825-1904). Science in the stable: or, how a horse can be kept in perfect health... **1894**. Easton, PA: Eschenbach. 87 pp. §
  Poor ventilation said to cause lameness.
955. **LUNGWITZ, A(nton)** (1845-). A text-book of horseshoeing, for horseshoers and veterinarians. Trans by J.W. Adams. **1904**. Phila: J.B. Lippincott. 216 pp. §
  A classic work on foot and shoeing.
956.__(same) **1913**. 11th ed, 216 pp. §
957.__; **ADAMS, John William** (1862-1926). (same) **1966**. Corvallis, OR: Oregon State Univ Press. 216 pp.

958. **LUPTON, James Irvine.** Horses: sound and unsound, with the law relating to sales and warranty. **1893.** London: Bailliere, Tindall. 211 pp.
   On warranty and trafficking in diseased animals.
959. **LYDEKKER, R.** The ox and its kindred. **1893.** London: Methuen. 271 pp. §
   Origin, domestication and types of cattle.
960. **(LYMAN, Charles Parker)** (1848-1918). The household physician: a twentieth century medica... **1924.** Buffalo: Brown-Flynn Publ Co. 1444 pp. §
   With 200-p veterinary dept by noted FRCVS.
961. **MAGNER, Dennis.** The art of taming and educating the horse: a system that makes easy and practical the subjection of wild and vicious horses... **1887.** Battle Creek, MI: Review & Herald Publ. 1088 pp.
   With large sections on shoeing and diseases.
962.__Facts for horse owners: a pictorial encyclopedia...including departments on shoeing, lameness, diseases, etc... **1894.** Battle Creek, MI: Magner Publ Co. 1216 pp. §
963.__Magner's A B C guide to sensible horseshoeing...including...methods of making a horse stand to be shod... **1899.** New York: Werner. 130 pp. §
   Mostly extracted from author's other works.
964.__Magner's standard horse and stock book: a complete...practical reference for horse and stock owners... **1887.** Battle Creek, MI: Review & Herald. 1080 pp. §
   On management and diseases, including dogs & cats.
965.__(same) **1906.** Akron, OH; Chicago: Saalfield Publ Co. 1181 pp. §
966.__(same) **1908.** 1181 pp.
967.__(same) **1911.** Chicago: Saalfield. 1181 pp.
968.__The new system of educating horses...feeding, watering, stabling, shoeing, etc...with practical treatment for diseases... **1870.** Buffalo: Warren, Johnson. 9th ed, 156 pp. §
969.__(same) **1876.** Rouses Point, NY: Lovell Printing & Publ. 11th ed, 226 pp.
970. **MAGRANE, William G.** A history of veterinary ophthalmology. **1988.** Elkhart, IN: Franklin Press. 76 pp. §
   With emphasis on contributions by individuals.
971. **MAHLICH, P.** Unsere Kaninchen. **1903.** Berlin: F. Pfenningstorff. 264 pp.
972. **MALKMUS, B(ernhard)** (1859-1925). Outlines of clinical diagnostics of the internal diseases of domestic animals. Trans by D.S. White & P. Fischer. **1904.** Chicago: A. Eger. 205 pp. §
   A long-time classic translated from German.
973.__(same) **1909.** 244 pp.
974.__(same) **1912.** 4th ed, 259 pp.
975. **MANNING, J. Russell.** The illustrated stock doctor and live-stock encyclopedia: including horses, cattle, sheep, swine and poultry... **1880?** Phila: Hubbard Bros. 1002 pp. §
   Offers treatment "without the aid of a professed veterinary surgeon," including use of anesthesia.
976.__(same) **1882.** Phila: Hubbard Bros; San Francisco: A.L Bancroft. 1082 pp. §

977.__Manning's horse book: comprising...breeds and their characteristics...general care, and all diseases to which they are subject... **1882**. Phila: Hubbard Bros. 516 pp. §

A generally sensible book for owners.

Gervase Markham (1568?-1637)

978.__ Cavalarice, or, the English horseman: contayning all the art of horsemanship... **1617**. [s.l. s.n.] 741 pp. §

A compilation by one with little knowledge of horses, including disease treatment.

979.__Cheap and good husbandry, for the well-ordering of all beasts and fowls, and for the general care of their diseases. **1664**. London: W. Wilson. 11th ed, 146 pp. §

A largely worthless but immensely popular work.

980.__Country contentments, or. the husbandmans recreations...hunting, hawking...bowling, tennis... **1654**. London: W. Wilson. 7th ed, 92 pp. §

For English gentlemen, taken from earlier works.

981.__Markham's farewell to husbandry, or, the enriching of all sorts of barren and sterile grounds... **1660**. London: G. Sawbridge. 126 pp.

Includes a short section on draft animals.

982.__Markhams maister-peece, or, what doth a horse-man lacke: containing all possible knowledge whatsoeuer which doth belong to any smith, farrier or horse-leech, touching the curing of all maner of sorrances in horses... **1610**. London: N. Okes. 502 pp. §

A retrograde compilation with many filthy and brutal remedies; the scarce first edition.

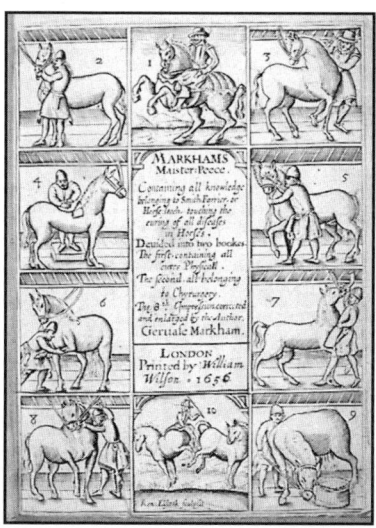

Markhams maister:peece, 1656 (983)

983.__Markhams maister:peece: containing all knowledge belonging to the smith, farrier, or horse-leech... **1656.** London: W. Wilson. 8th ed, 591 pp. §

Went through 21 editions; "...no work...has done more damage to veterinary progress." (Smith)

984.__ The perfect horse-man, or, the experienced secrets of Mr. Markham's fifty years practice... **1671.** London: R. Chiswell. The last edition, 175 pp. §

"A horrible book...evidence of the low taste of public knowledge." (Smith) Posthumous work.

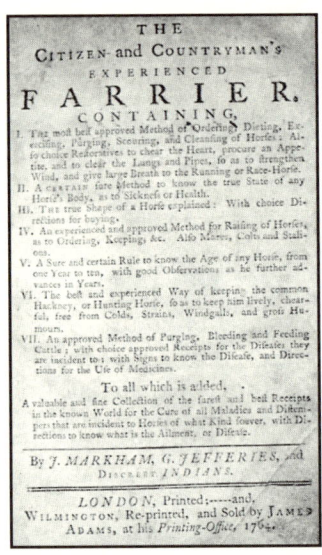

Markham and Jefferies: 1764 (985)

985. **MARKHAM, J. (Gervase); JEFFERIES, G(reg) and Discreet Indians.** The citizen and countryman's experienced farrier...to all which is added...the surest and best receipts...for the cure of all maladies and distempers that are incident to horses... **1764.** London, Printed; Wilmington, DE, Reprinted: James Adams. 364 pp. §

American imprint based on Markhams maister-peece.

986.__(same) **1797.** Baltimore: S. Sower. 349 pp. §

987. **MARKHAM; JEFFERIES and Experienced Indians.** (same) 1803. 349 pp. §

988.__(same) **1839.** Chambersburg, PA: T.J. Wright. 332 pp. §

989. **MARSH, Charles Dwight** (1855-1932). The loco-weed disease of the plains. **1909.** Washington: GPO. 130 pp. §

A study of locoism in horses, cattle and sheep.

990. **MARSHALL, F(rancis) H(ugh) A(dam)** (1878-1949). The physiology of reproduction. **1910.** London; New York: Longmans, Green. 706 pp. §

A classic comparative text; includes lactation.

991. **MASCALL, Leonard D.** (-1589). The first booke of cattell: wherein is shewn the gouernment of oxen, kine, calues...with diuerse and approued remedies to helpe most diseases among cattell... **1591.** London: printed by J. Wolfe. 296 pp. §
   A thoroughly retrograde plagiarized work.

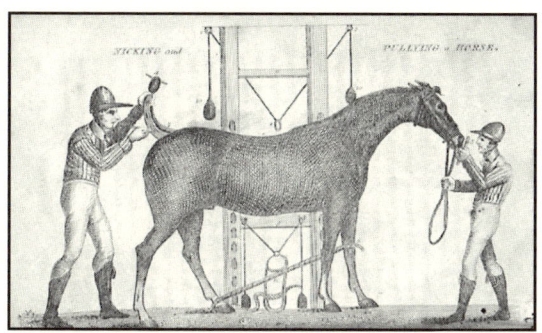

Mason: The gentleman's new pocket farrier, 1825 (992)

992. **MASON, Richard.** The gentleman's new pocket farrier...also, a concise account of the diseases to which the horse is subject... **1825.** Richmond, VA: P. Cottom. 3rd ed, 228 pp.
   A practical handbook for farmers and horsemen.
993. __(same) **1830.** 5th ed, 388 pp. §
994. __(same) **1844.** Phila: Grigg & Elliot. 8th ed, 419 pp. §
995. __(same) **1847.** 419 pp. §
996. __(same) **1851.** Phila: Lippincott, Grambo. 415 + 101 pp.
997. __(same) **1856.** Phila: J.B. Lippincott. 415 + 101 pp. §
   With appendix on mules by J.S. Skinner.
998. __(same) **1857.** §
999.(__) Mason's farrier and cattle book: comprising a general description of the horse...with treatment in disease...to which is added a prize essay on mules. **1885.** New York: Hurst & Co. 314 pp. §
   Without Annals of the turf, as in early editions.
1000. __The practical farrier, for farmers: comprising a general description of...the horse...with treatment in disease... **1860.** Phila: J.B. Lippincott. 288 pp.
1001. **MAXWELL, Robert** (1695-1765). The practical husbandman: being a collection of miscellaneous papers on husbandry. **1757.** The author. 430 pp.
   An early work on improvement of agriculture.
1002. **MAYER, John.** The sportsman's directory...containing instructions for breeding, feeding, and breaking dogs... **1819.** London: Baldwin, Craddock. 3rd ed, 204 pp.
1003. **MAYHEW, Edward** (1813?-1868). Dogs: their management. Being a new plan of treating the animal, based upon a consideration of his natural temperament. **1854.** London: G. Routledge. 264 pp. §
   Urges paying more attention to canine disease.

1004.__The illustrated horse doctor: being an...account of the various diseases to which the equine race are subjected, together with the latest mode of treatment... **1861.** New York: D. Appleton. 536 pp.

An excellent work by an experienced veterinarian.

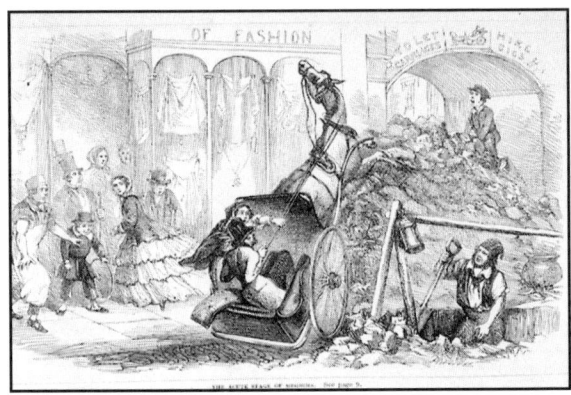

Mayhew: The illustrated horse doctor, 1864 (1005)

1005.__(same) **1864.** London: W.H. Allen. 4th ed, 592 pp. §

1006.__(same) **1887.** New York: D. Appleton. 610 pp.

With additions on influenza and shoeing.

1007.__(same) **1888.** Phila: J.B. Lippincott. 522 pp.

Similar to 1861 edition.

1008.__The illustrated horse management: containing descriptive remarks upon anatomy, medicine, shoeing, teeth, food, vices, stables... **1865.** Phila: J.B. Lippincott. 548 pp. §

1009.__(same) **1901.** London: W. Glaisher. 17th ed, 356 pp. §

1010. **MAYO, Nelson Slater** (1866-). The diseases of animals: a book of brief and popular advice... **1913.** New York: Macmillan. 8th ed, 459 pp. §

A better-than-average farmer's handbook.

1011. **MAZZA, Vincenzo.** Sul moccio del cavallo detto impropriamente morva...dei corpi di cavalleria. **1841.** Napoli: G. Palma. 234 pp.

On infectious diseases of horses.

1012. **M'CRUM, William B.** The horseman's friend, or, pocket counselor. **1869.** Fort Wayne, IN: Daily Gazette. 22 pp. §

A worthless collection of remedies.

1013. **MacCALLUM, Alexander Inglis.** The horse in health and in disease...structure and functions of the various systems and their more common ailments... **1910.** Edinburgh: Livingstone & Logan. 87 pp.

Includes diseases communicable to man.

1014. **McCLURE, Robert.** American horse, cattle and sheep doctor. **1870.** Phila: Porter & Cable. 413 pp.

A mediocre work in dictionary form.

1015.__Diseases in the American stable, field & farmyard: containing...the most approved methods of treatment, and the properties and use of remedies... **1866.** Phila: The author. 414 pp. §
 Said to be based on lectures at Phila Vet Coll.
1016.__Diseases of the American horse, and cattle and sheep. Their treatment, with...the medicines employed. **1870.** Phila: J.E. Potter. 413 pp. §
 Essentially the same as item 1014.
1017.__The gentleman's stable guide: containing a familiar description of the American stable...and general management of horses... **1870.** Phila: Porter & Coates. 184 pp. §
 A sensible work on stable management.
1018.(__) McClure's American horse, cattle and sheep doctor... **1917.** Chicago: F.J. Drake. 413 pp. §
 Identical to item 1016.
1019.__; **WALSH. J.H., et al.** Every horse owner's cyclopedia: the anatomy and physiology of the horse...diseases and how to cure them... **1871.** Phila: Porter & Coates. 582 pp. §
 About 95% of book is from Walsh: The horse (qv).
1020. **McCULLOUGH, Laurence B.; MORRIS, James P.** (eds). Implications of history and ethics to medicine—veterinary and human. **1978.** College Station: Texas A&M Univ. 158 pp. §
 The proceedings of a symposium at Texas A&M.
1021. **McEACHRAN, Duncan McNab** (1841-1924); **SMITH, Andrew D.** (-1914). The Canadian horse and his diseases. **1867.** Toronto: J. Campbell. 219 pp. §
 By two noted Canadian veterinary educators.
1022. **McFADYEAN, John, Sir** (1853-1941). The anatomy of the horse: a dissection guide. **1884.** New York: W.R. Jenkins. 375 pp.
 A detailed work with numerous illustrations.
1023.__(same) **1908.** 388 pp. §
1024.__(same) **1909.** 2nd ed, 388 pp.
1025. **McFARLAND, Joseph** (1868-1945). A text-book upon the pathogenic bacteria, for students of medicine and physicians. **1906.** Phila; London: W.B. Saunders. 5th ed, 647 pp.
 Includes several common zoonoses.
1026. **McGOWAN, John Pool.** On rous, leukotic & allied tumours in the fowl. A study in malignancy. **1928.** New York: Macmillan. 99 pp.
 An early work on avian tumors.
1027. **McINTOSH, Donald.** Diseases of horses and cattle ...for the farmer, stockman and veterinary student. **1895.** Chicago: M.A. Donohue. 390 pp.
 Generally acceptable; detailed plates of calving.
1028.__Diseases of swine...for the veterinary surgeon, student and swine grower. **1897.** Chicago: M.A. Donohue. 230 pp.
 Ill-suited for primary audience.
1029. **(MEDICINE).** Nature the best physician, or every man his own doctor... **1735.** London: J. Cooke. 71 pp.

74   *Five Centuries of Veterinary Medicine*

1030.__Primer on fractures. **1931.** Chicago: Amer Med Assn. 2nd ed, 63 pp.
   Diagnosis and treatment; E.A. Ehmer signature.
1031. **MELLEN, Ida M.** The science and mystery of the cat: its evolutionary status...so-called "occult powers," and its effect on people. **1949.** New York: Scribners. 275 pp. §
   Includes physiology, psychology and behavior.
1032. **MERILLAT, Louis Adolph** (1868-1956). Fistula of the withers and poll-evil. **1917.** Chicago: Am Vet Publ Co. 138 pp. §
   Cause and treatment of a common problem.
1033.__Veterinary surgery, vol 1. Animal dentistry and diseases of the mouth. **1905.** Chicago: A. Eger. 261 pp. §
   Details of tooth structure and diseases.
1034.__Veterinary surgery, vol 2. The principles of veterinary surgery. **1906.** Chicago: A. Eger. 669 pp. §
   A general text including restraint and anesthesia.
1035.__(same) **1915.** 2nd ed, 352 pp. §
1036.__Veterinary surgery, vol 3. Veterinary surgical operations. **1909.** Chicago: A. Eger. 521 pp. §
   Indications and technic for numerous procedures.
1037.__(same) **1912.** 521 pp. §
1038.__(same) **1921.** 2nd ed, 556 pp. §
1039.__; **CAMPBELL, D(elwyn) M(orton)** (1880-). Veterinary military history of the United States: with a brief record of the development of veterinary education, practice, organization and legislation. **1935.** Chicago: Vet Magazine Co. 2 vol, 620; 652 pp. §
   A discursive history from late 1700s, with civilian matters interspersed.
1040. **METCHNIKOFF, Elie** (1845-1916). The founders of modern medicine: Pasteur, Koch, Lister. **1939.** New York: Walden. 387 pp. §
   With extracts of writings on infection, rabies, etc.
1041. **MEYER, F.** Abhandlung uber die Pferde-influenza, auch Brustfell oder Lungenentzundung gennant... **1841.** Potsdam: The author. 48 pp.
   On control of equine influenza.
1042. **MEYSEY-THOMPSON, Richard Frederick** (1847-). The horse, its origin and development combined with stable practice. **1911.** London: E. Arnold. 436 pp.
   With a section of dubious value on diseases.
1043. **MICHELS, John** (1875-). Dairy farming. **1908.** West Raleigh: NC: The author. 2nd ed, 212 pp.
   A basic work for students and farmers.
1044. **(MICHIGAN).** Annual report...State Board of Agriculture... **1867.** Lansing, MI: J.A. Kerr. 496 pp. §
   Articles on sheep breeding and cattle disease.
1045. **MIESSNER, Hermann** (1870-). Epizootics and their control during war: a guide for army, government and practicing veterinarians. Trans by A.A. Leipold. **1917.** Chicago: Amer Vet Publ Co. 215 pp. §

1046. **MILES, Manly** (1826-1898). Stock-breeding: a practical treatise on the application of the laws of development and heredity to the improvement...of domestic animals. **1888.** New York: D. Appleton. 428 pp. §

1047. **MILES, William.** The horse's foot and how to keep it sound. **1847.** New York: D. Appleton; Phila: G.S. Appleton. 70 pp. §

A practical work based largely on work of others.

1048.__(same) **1847.** London: Longman, Brown; Exeter: H.J. Wallis & W. Spreat. 5th ed, 90 pp. §

Appendix on shoeing added; detailed plates.

1049.__On horseshoeing. **1858.** Boston: J.H. Eastburn's Press. 27 pp. §

Reprint of a nontechnical journal article.

1050.__Modern practical farriery...a complete system of the veterinary art, as at present practiced at the Royal Veterinary College, London. **1874?** London: William Mackenzie. 536 + 96 pp.

With sections by other writers; numerous plates.

1051.__(same) **1892?** 536 pp.

1052.__(same) **1892?** In 5 vol, 641 pp. §

1053. **MILKS, Howard Jay** (1879-). Practical veterinary pharmacology and therapeutics. **1917.** New York: Macmillan. 518 pp. §

First ed; some sections unchanged for 30 years.

1054.__Practical veterinary pharmacology, materia medica and therapeutics. **1930.** Chicago: A. Eger. 2nd ed, 539 pp. §

With chapter on biologics by A. Eichhorn.

1055.__(same) **1943.** 5th ed, 673 pp. §

1056. **MILLER, Everett B.** United States Army Veterinary Service in World War II. **1961.** Washington: Office of the Surgeon General. 779 pp. §

Includes history of Army Veterinary Service.

1057. **MILLER, William B.E.; TELLOR, Lloyd V.** The diseases of livestock and their most efficient remedies...giving in brief...the most successful treatment of American, English and European veterinarians. **1885.** Phila: H.C. Watts. 523 pp. §

Identical to Tellor (1881) with diseases of dogs and poultry added.

1058.__(same) **1900.** Phila: D. McKay. 523 pp. §

1059. **MILLS, John** (-1784). The modern system of farriery: shewing the most approved methods of breeding, rearing, and fitting for use, all kinds of horses...with treatment of them in their several disorders. **1796.** Boston: William Spottswood. 274 pp.

Reprint of British work by a near-ignoramus.

1060.__A treatise on cattle: shewing the most approved methods of breeding, rearing and fitting for use, asses, mules, horned cattle, sheep, goats, and swine...with treatment of...disorders... **1776.** London: J. Johnson: 498 pp.

Largely worthless; G.E. Fussell signature.

1061.__(same) **1795.** Boston: William Spottswood: 216 pp. §

1062. **MILLS, Wesley** (1847-1915). The dog in health and in disease, including his origin, history...education, and general management in health, and his treatment in disease. **1892.** New York: D. Appleton. 407 pp.

Written for owners and veterinary students.

1063.__(same) **1901**. 408 pp. §
1064.__(same) **1916**. 2nd ed, 408 pp.
1065. **MINERE, Th.** Osteolymphatisme du cheval de course et nouvelle methode d'exercice et d'entrainement. **1914**. Paris: J.-B. Bailliere. 640 pp. §
   On an obscure bone disease of racehorses.
1066. **MITCHELL, C.A.** A note on the early history of veterinary science in Canada. **1940**. Gardenvale, Que: Natl Business Publ. 48 pp. §
1067. **MITCHELL-VIGNERON, Jeanette.** Alexandre Liautard (1835-1918) Sa vie—son oeuvre. These pour le doctorat veterinaire. **1982**. Alfort: L'Ecole Nationale Veterinaire. 85 pp. §
   Biography of A. Liautard, noted American vet educator. Inscribed by author to J.F. Smithcors.
1068. **MOHR, John H.** Medical guide in treating all internal and external diseases of horses, mules and neat cattle. **1868**. Reading, PA: Owen's Press. 262 pp.
   A Penna-German work; remedies in English & German.
1069. **MOLLER, Heinrich** (1841-1932). Die Hufkrankheiten des Pferdes, ihre Erkennung, Heilung und Verhutung. **1880**. Berlin: Wiegandt, Hempel. 260 pp.
   Diagnosis and treatment of equine foot diseases.
1070.__Lehrbuch der speciellen Chirurgie fur Thierarzte. **1891**. Stuttgart: F. Enke. 872 pp.
   A comprehensive surgery of domestic animals.
1071.__(same) **1893**. 2nd ed, 872 pp.
1072.__Moller's operative veterinary surgery. Trans by Jno A.W. Dollar. **1899**. New York: W.R. Jenkins. 773 pp.
   From the 1894 German edition.
1073.__(same) **1902**. 733 pp.
1074.__; **DOLLAR, John A(rchibald) W(att).** Regional veterinary surgery. **1904**. New York: W.R. Jenkins. 853 pp. §
   An expanded version of item 1072.
1075.__(same) **1906**. 853 pp.
1076.__(same) **1908**. 853 pp.
1077.__(same) **1909**. 853 pp. §
1078. **MONTANE, Lucien; BOURDELLE, E.; BRESSOU, C.J.P.** Anatomie regionale des animaux domestiques. 4 vol. 1913-1953. Paris: J.-B. Bailliere. Vol 1. Equides: cheval -ane - mulet. **1913**. 1069 pp. §
   A detailed anatomy, with histology & embryology.
1079.__Vol 2 (Montane et Bourdelle). Ruminants. **1917**. 384 pp. §
   Inscribed to L.A. Merillat by Bourdelle.
1080.__Vol 3 (Bourdelle). Porc. **1920**. 365 pp. §
   Inscribed to L.A. Merillat by Bourdelle.
1081.__Vol 2 & 3 bound together.
1082.__(same) **1937**. (Bourdelle et Bressou.) 2nd ed. Vol 1, fasc. 2. Tete et encolare. 469 pp.
1083.__Vol 4 (Bourdelle et Bressou). Carnivores: Chien et Chat. **1953**. 502 pp. §

1084. **MONVOISIN, A.** Precis de diagnostic veterinaire. **1929.** Paris: Vigot Freres. 2nd ed, 472 pp. §
   On physical diagnosis and laboratory methods.

1085. **MOORE, James.** Common diseases of animals and their homoeopathic treatment... **1859.** Manchester: H. Turner. 126 pp. §
   Abridged from author's "Outlines..." (item 1088).

1086.___The diseases of dogs and their homoeopathic treatment. **1863.** London: Simpkin, Marshall. 320 pp. §
   An early canine homeopathy for owners.

1087.___Horses ill and well: homoeopathic treatment of diseases and injuries and hints on feeding...etc. **1875.** London: James Epps. 2nd ed, 220 pp. §
   With a materia medica indexed to diseases.

1088.___Outlines of veterinary homoeopathy: comprising horse, cow, dog, sheep and hog diseases... **1871.** 6th ed, 295 pp.
   Gives 3-6 treatments for each disease.

1089. **MOORE, Robert C.** (1852-). Interrogatory surgery for students of veterinary science. **1904.** Kansas City: The author. 284 pp.
   Questions keyed to Moller's operative surgery.

1090. **MOORE, Veranus Alva** (1859-1931). Cornstalk disease, and rabies in cattle... **1896.** Washington: GPO. 92 pp. §
   An early report on a rabies-like disease.

1091.___New York State Veterinary College, a special report to the president of Cornell University. **1908.** Ithaca, NY: Cornell Univ. 36 pp. §
   Outlines the needs of the veterinary college.

1092.___The pathology and differential diagnosis of infectious diseases of animals... **1916.** New York: Macmillan. 4th ed, 577 pp.
   A standard text for students and practitioners.

1093.___Veterinary education and service at Cornell University 1896-1929. **1929.** [s.l. s.n.] 243 pp. §
   The faculty, research work and publications.

1094. **MOORE, William; FAULHABER, L.J.; BROWN, J.M.** A veterinary history of North Carolina. **1946.** New Bern, NC: O.G. Dunn. 108 pp. §
   Includes lists of NC veterinarians.

1095. **MORRELL, Luke A.** The American shepherd: being a history of the sheep, with their breeds, management, and diseases... **1845.** New York: Harper. 437 pp. §
   Section on diseases is brief but sensible.

1096.___(same) **1854.** 437 pp. §

1097. **MORRILL, Charles Cleon** (1907-). Veterinary medicine in Michigan: an illustrated history. **1979.** East Lansing: Mich State Univ. 178 pp.
   From before 1850, with emphasis on education; many plates from MSU vet history collection.

1098. **MORTON, William John Thomas** (1800-1868). A manual of pharmacy for the student of veterinary medicine: containing the substances employed at the Royal Veterinary College...and the pharmacopoeia of that institution. **1860.** London: Longman, Green. 6th ed, 544 pp. §
   Includes medications for large and small animals.

1099.__(same) **1868.** 7th ed, 544 pp. §

1100. **MOSSELMAN, Gustave; DOLLAR, Jno. A.W.** Diseases of cattle, sheep, goats and swine. **1905.** New York: W.R. Jenkins. 785 pp.

From French, German and British sources.

1101.__; **LINAUX, E.** Manual of veterinary microbiology. Trans by R.R. Dinwiddie. **1895.** New York: W.R. Jenkins. 342 pp.

A student text, translated from French.

1102. **MOUSSU, Gustave** (1864-). Les principales maladies des habitants de la basse-cour... **1942.** Paris: Maison Rustique. 4th ed, 355 pp. §

Diseases of poultry and rabbits.

1103. **MUIR, Robert, Sir** (1864-1959). Manual of bacteriology. Rev from 3rd English ed by N.M. Harris. **1905.** New York; London: Macmillan. 565 pp.

A general text, including several zoonoses.

1104. **MULLER, Georg Alfred** (1851-1923). Die Krankheiten des Hundes und ihre Behandlung. **1892.** Berlin: P. Parey. 433 pp.

An early classic on diseases of the dog.

1105.__; **GLASS, Alexander.** Diseases of the dog and their treatment. **1909.** Chicago: A. Eger. 419 pp. §

A long-standard translation used in the US.

1106.__(same) **1912.** 3rd ed, 506 pp. §

1107.__(same) **1922.** 4th ed, 506 pp. §

1108.__(same) **1926.** 625 pp. §

With J.V. Lacroix signature.

1109. **MUMFORD, F.B.** History of the Missouri College of Agriculture. **1944.** Columbia, MO: The College. 300 pp. §

Includes brief mention of veterinary science.

1110. **MUNRO, John McKenzie.** The complete horse doctor and cattle cure collection: being a thorough treatise on all diseases incident to horses and cattle... **1881.** San Francisco: [s.n.] 237 pp. §

Badly written by an uneducated practitioner.

1111. **MURRAY, Alexander James.** Cattle and their diseases...with an introduction on the breeding and management of cattle... **1890.** Chicago: J.H. Sanders. 270 pp. §

A generally sensible compilation for farmers.

1112. **MURRAY, W(illiam) H(enry) H(arrison)** (1840-1904). The perfect horse: how to know him...Intro by Rev. Henry Ward Beecher... **1873.** Boston: J.R. Osgood. 480 pp.

A discursive work by a clergyman, with a section on shoeing largely from Fleming and Lafosse.

1113. **MURRAY, Charles.** History of veterinary medicine in Iowa, **1957-58.** Iowa Veterinarian, Vol 28, Nos. 4-6; Vol 29, No. 1. §

Education, practice and association matters.

1114. **(MUSEUMS).** The museum of veterinary history at Skara. **1981.** Skara, Sweden: [s.n.] 7 pp. §

1115.__Stuhr Museum of the Prairie Pioneer. A century of veterinary medicine in Nebraska. **1986.** Grand Island, NE: Prairie Pioneer Press. 20 pp. §
   With details of reconstructed early vet hospital.
1116. **MYERS, J(ay) Arthur** (1888-1978). Man's greatest victory over tuberculosis. **1940.** Springfield, IL; Baltimore: Charles C. Thomas. 419 pp. §
   Details veterinary achievements in control of TB.
1117.__Tuberculosis among children and young adults... **1938.** Springfield, IL; Baltimore: Charles C. Thomas. 401 pp.
   Includes references to TB testing in cattle.
1118. **NAKAMURA, Yokichi.** [Veterinary history of Japan] **1980.** In Japanese. 295 pp. §
   With letter from author to J.F. Smithcors.
1119. **NASH, Ephraim.** The farmer's practical horse farriery: containing Rarey's art of taiming [sic] vicious horses, with...symptoms, treatment and cure of diseases... **1857.** Auburn, NY: The author. 197 pp. §
   Largely from other sources, eg, Rarey (qv).
1120.__(same) **1858.** 197 pp. §
1121. **NAVIN, John Nicholson.** Navin's veterinary practice: or explanatory horse doctor... **1868.** Indianapolis: Roach & Thistlethwaite. 506 pp. §
   Mediocre; promotes bloodletting as a cure-all.
1122.__(same) **1869.** 506 pp.
1123.__(same) **1873.** 506 pp.
1124.__(same) **1873.** Indianapolis: John B. Hahn. Bound with Part 2. A practical treatise on the diseases of cattle, hogs, sheep, and poultry. 506 + 229 pp. §
1125. **NEUMANN, Louis Georges** (1846-). A treatise on the parasites and parasitic diseases of the domesticated animals. Trans by George Fleming. **1892.** London: Bailliere, Tindall. 800 pp. §
   A classic work translated from French.
1126.__(same) Rev by James MacQueen. **1905.** 677 pp.
1127. **NEVERS, Philippe Julien** (1641-1707). Le parfait cocher...avec des principales maladies, auxquelles les chevaux... **1744.** Paris: P.G. Merigot. 373 pp. §
   On coaching, with maladies of coach horses.
1128. **NEWSHOLME, Arthur, Sir** (1857-1943). Fifty years in public health: a personal narrative with comments. **1935.** London: Allen & Unwin. 415 pp. §
   Includes milk hygiene and bovine tuberculosis.
1129. **NICHOLAS, Eugene** (1867-). Veterinary and comparative ophthalmology... Trans by Henry Gray. **1930.** London: H. & W. Brown. 598 pp. §
1130. **NIGHTINGALE, Florence** (1820-1910). Notes on nursing. **1860.** New York: D. Appleton. 140 pp.
   A classic work by founder of modern nursing.
1131. **NIMROD (Col Charles James Apperley)** (1779-1843). The chace, the road and the turf. Intro by W. Shaw Sparrow. **1927.** London: John Lane. 231 pp. §
   On 19thC hunting and racing in England.

1132.__Remarks on the condition of hunters, the choice of horses, and their management. **1834.** London: M.A. Pittman. 2nd ed, 503 pp. §

Sensible writing by a first-class horseman and friend of the veterinary profession.

1133.__(same) **1837.** 3rd ed, 503 pp. §

NOLAN, L.E.—see Garrard, K.

1134. **OEYNHAUSEN, R. von.** Der Pferdeliebhaber: ein handbuch uber Pferdekenntnis in weiteren Sinne... **1865.** Wien: L.W. Seidel. 418 pp.

A handbook for horse owners.

1135. **OFFUTT, Denton.** The educated horse: teaching horses and other animals to obey...also, breeding of animals... **1854.** Washington: [s.n.] 308 pp. §

Horse taming, equine diseases and moral doctrine.

1136. **O'HANLON, Jeremiah.** The horse and its diseases. **1864.** Cork, Ireland: Henry & Coughlan. 172 pp. §

Of interest for observations on Irish practice.

1137. **(OHIO).** Report of the Ohio State Board of Agriculture for the year 1857. **1858.** Columbus: Richard Nevins. 823 pp. §

Reports on hog cholera, cattle diseases, etc.

1138. **ORFILA, Matthieu Joseph** (1787-1853). Lecons de toxicologie. **1858.** Paris: Labe. 120 pp. §

Primarily on arsenic poisoning.

1139. **OSLER, William, Sir** (1849-1919). The principles and practice of medicine: designed for use of practitioners and students of medicine. **1894.** New York: D. Appleton. 1079 pp. §

A classic work, including diseases caused by animal parasites, and other zoonoses.

1140. **OSMER, William.** A treatise on diseases and lameness of horses. **1759.** London: T. Waller. 125 pp.

A curious work, dealt with at length by Smith.

1141. **OSTERTAG, Robert von** (1864-1940). Handbook of meat inspection. Trans by E.V. Wilcox. **1905.** New York: W.R. Jenkins. 2nd ed, 884 pp. §

Translation of a classic German work.

1142.__(same) **1907.** 3rd ed, 884 pp.

1143. **OWEN, Richard** (1804-1892). Lectures on the comparative anatomy and physiology of the vertebrate animals...Part I: Fishes. **1846.** London: Longman, Brown. 308 pp. §

1144. **(PACKER, R. Allen, et al).** The first 100 years of the College of Veterinary Medicine, Iowa State University: a pictorial history. **1981?** Ames, IA: Iowa State Univ. 190 pp.

Remarkable photos of faculty, students, ISU.

1145. **PAGE, Charles Edward** (1840-). Horses: their feed and their feet. A manual of horse hygiene... **1883.** New York: Fowler & Wells. 171 pp. §

Of little utility, by an amateur.

1146. **PAMMEL, L.** The manual of poisonous plants. **1911.** Cedar Rapids, IA: Torch Press. 977 pp. §

A copiously illustrated taxonomic work.

1147. **PARENT. Ernest** (1835). Le livre de toutes les chasse. Vol 1. **1865.** Paris: C. Tanera. 172 pp. §
   A dictionary of hunting.
1148. **PARKINSON, Richard** (1748-1815). Treatise on the breeding and management of live stock... **1810.** London: Cadell & Davies. 2 vol, 436; 484 pp. §
   For owners; worthless section on diseases.
1149. **PARKINSON, Thomas.** A treatise on the management of parturient animals. **1812.** Nottingham: H. Barnett. 118 pp. §
   A enlightened work by an expert with sheep.
1150. **PARSONS, John Herbert, Sir** (1868-). Diseases of the eye. **1930.** New York: Macmillan. 678 pp.
   A comprehensive human text.
1151. **(PASTEUR, Louis)** (1822-1895). Correspondence of Pasteur and Thuillier concerning anthrax and swine fever vaccinations. Trans by R.M. Frank & Denise Wrotnowska. **1969.** University, AL: Univ Alabama Press. 240 pp. §
   Previously unpublished details of research.
1152. **(PATENTS).** Report of the commissioner of patents for 1853. **1854.** Washington: B. Tucker. 448 pp. §
   Short history of early animal imports; C.T. Jackson's claim of rediscovery of anesthesia.
1153. __(same)...for 1859: agriculture. **1860.** Washington: G.W. Bowman. 590 pp. §
   Articles on vet education; animal disease.
1154. __(same)...for 1860: agriculture. **1861.** Washington: GPO. 504 pp. §
   Includes section on bovine pleuropneumonia.
1155. **PATER, Erra.** The compleat and experienced farrier and cowleech. [Photocopy extract from] The book of knowledge...Trans by W. Lilly. **1794.** Canaan, NY: T. Spencer. pp 75-88. §
   Remedies based on superstition and magic.
1156. **PATON, Diarmid Noel** (1859-1828). Essentials of physiology for veterinary students. **1908.** Chicago: W.T. Keener. 2nd ed, 464 pp. §
   A copiously illustrated text.
1157. **PATTISON, Ian** (1914-). John McFadyean: a great British veterinarian. **1981.** London; New York: J.A. Allen. 240 pp.
   The "father" of veterinary research in Britain.
1158. **PATTON, Charles U.** The common-sense horse book, being a clear and comprehensive treatment of all diseases...also, the most sensible mode of taming...the horse. **1875.** Cincinnati: Mecklenborg. 128 pp. §
   Mediocre, with "directions for new liniments."
1159. **PEALL, Thomas.** Observations...on some of the more common diseases of the horse...diet, and the ordinary stable management of that animal. **1814.** Cork, Ireland: J. Bolster. 352 pp. §
   An enlightened and informative work.
1160. **(PEARSON, Leonard)** (1868-1909). In memoriam: Leonard Pearson...State Veterinarian...Dean of Veterinary College of University of Pennsylvania... **1910.** [s.l. s.n.] 103 pp. §
   A biography and memorial tributes.

1161.__; **WARREN, Benjamin Harry** (1858-). Diseases and enemies of poultry... **1897**. Harrisburg, PA: C.M. Busch. 731 pp. §
 With fine color plates of predators.
1162. **PECK, W.** Veterinary medicine, and therapeutics: containing...the symptoms, cause and treatment of diseases... **1814**. London: Newman & Co. 175 pp. §
 Good pharmacopoeia, poor on diseases.
1163. **PELLERIN, C.** Median neurotomy in the treatment of chronic tendinitis and periostitis of the fetlock. Trans by A. Liautard. **1896**. New York: W.R. Jenkins. 61 pp.
 By a pioneer of the technic; trans from French.
1164. **PEMBROKE, Henry Herbert, Earl of** (1734-1794). Military equitation: or, A method of breaking horses, and teaching soldiers to ride... **1793**. London: G. & T. Wilkie. 4th ed, 140 pp. §
 Includes sections on shoeing and management.
1165. **(PENNSYLVANIA)**. Second annual report of the Pennsylvania Department of Agriculture. **1896**. Harrisburg, PA: The Dept. 820 pp. §
 With reports on rabies and other diseases.
1166. **PERCIVALL, William** (1793-1854). The anatomy of the horse, embracing the structure of the foot. **1858**. London: Longman, Brown. 455 pp.
 The first (1832) equine anatomy text in English.
1167.__(same) **1868**. Longmans, Green. 455 pp. §

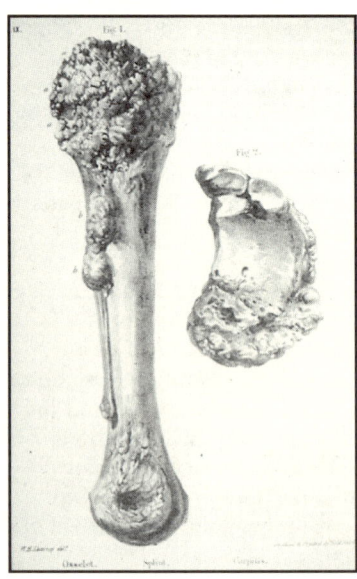

Percivall: Lameness in the horse. Part 1,
vol. iv of the Hippopathology, 1849
(1168)

1168.___Hippopathology: a systematic treatise on the disorders and lameness of the horse: with their modern and most approved methods of cure... **1834-52.** London: Longman, Rees. 4 vol in 5 parts; 331; 428; 358; (vol 4) 271; 514 pp. §

"The best exposition of medical and surgical practice ever published...a contribution to English literature." (Smith)

1169.___(same) **1853-76.** London: Longmans, Green. 2nd ed. 4 vol in 6 parts; 307; 592; 358; 514 pp.

1170.___A series of elementary lectures on the veterinary art...the anatomy, physiology, and pathology of the horse... **1823-26.** London: J. Hill. 3 vol, 377; 377; 502 pp. §

A highly original work, based on experience.

1171. **PERRIAM, Jonathan.** The groundswell. A history of the origin, aims, and progress of the farmers' movement... **1874.** Cincinnati: E. Hannaford. 576 pp.

An exhaustive study of a complex subject.

1172.___The prairie farmer horse book...care and management...diseases and remedies... **1891.** Chicago: Prairie Farmer Publ Co. 347 pp.

With observations on soundness and heredity.

1173.___; **BAKER, Arthur Hart** (1852-). The American farmer's pictorial cyclopedia of live stock...being also a complete stock doctor... **1884.** St Louis; New York: N.D. Thompson. 1246 pp. §

A generally useful omnibus volume for owners.

1174.___The new pictorial cyclopedia of live stock...[and] stock doctor... **1902.** St Louis: N.D. Thompson. 1438 pp.

Essentially identical to 1884 edition.

1175.___Live stock: a complete compendium for the farmer and stock owner...also a complete stock doctor... **1910.** St Louis: N.D. Thompson. 1298 pp.

Like 1902 ed, but without section on dogs.

1176. **PERRY, Joseph Franklin** ("Ashmont"). Dogs: their management and treatment in disease: a study of the theory and practice of canine medicine. **1885.** Boston: J.L. Thayer. 204 pp. §

Little on management but good on disease.

1177.___(same) **1891.** 2nd ed, 221 pp. §

1178.___Kennel diseases: their symptoms, nature, causes and treatment. **1921.** Boston: Little, Brown. 424 pp. §

An improved version of the author's earlier work.

1179.___Kennel secrets: how to breed, exhibit and manage dogs. **1916.** Boston: Little, Brown. Rev ed, 344 pp. §

A comprehensive work for kennel owners.

1180. **PETTIGREW, Thomas Joseph** (1791-1865). On superstitions connected with the history and practice of medicine and surgery. **1844.** London: J. Churchill. 167 pp. §

Alchemy, astrology, charms, quackery, etc.

1181. **PEUCH, F.; TOUSSAINT, H.** Precis de chirurgie veterinaire: comprenant l'anatomie chirurgicale et la medecine operatoire. **1876-77.** Paris: P. Asselin. 2 vol, 696; 845 pp. §

Mainly equine surgery; L.A. Merillat signature.

1182. (PHARMACOPOEIA). Veterinair-pharmacopoe. **1890.** Kjobehavn: Glydendalske Boghandels. 56 pp.
    A Danish pharmacopoeia and materia medica.
1183. (PHILADELPHIA SOCIETY). Memoirs of the Philadelphia Society for Promoting Agriculture. **1808-18.** Phila: J. Aitken. Vol 1 (1808), 331 pp; Vol 2 (1811), 362 pp; Vol 3 (1814), 440 pp; Vol 4 (1818), 332 pp. §
    Includes "veterinary essay" by Benjamin Rush (vol 1) and many items of veterinary interest.
1184. **PHILLIPS, Paul C(hrisler)** (1883-1956). Medicine in the making of Montana. **1962.** Missoula: Montana Med Assn. 564 pp.
1185. **PICARD, Madge E.; BULEY, R. Carlyle.** The midwest pioneer, his ills, cures, & doctors. **1946.** New York: H. Schuman. 339 pp. §
    Frontier medicine; some items on animal disease.
1186. **PIRES, Antonio.** Tratado de las enfermedades del pie del caballo. **1949.** Buenos Aires: Guillermo Kraft. 351 pp. §
    On equine foot diseases, with extensive topical references; inscribed to J.G. Hardenbergh (AVMA).
1187. **PITCHER, B.** Das Pferd. Ein buch fur das volk... **1881.** Chicago: The author. 3rd ed, 177 pp.
    On horse management and diseases, with remedies.
1188. **PLINY, the Elder** (23-69 AD). The historie of the world: commonly called, The naturall historie of C. Plinivs Secundus. Trans by Philemon Holland (1601). **1634.** London: A. Islip. 2 vol in 1; 614; 632 pp. §
    An omnibus work; many items of vet interest.
1189. **PLUMB, Charles Sumner** (1860-1939). Types and breeds of farm animals. **1906.** Boston: Ginn. 563 pp.
    A long-popular textbook on the subject.
1190. **PORTER, James Amos** (1905-). Doctor, spare my cow! **1956.** Ames, IA: Iowa State Univ Press. 238 pp. §
    Experiences with the Mexican foot-and-mouth disease outbreak 1947-52.
1191. **PORTSMOUTH, Gerard V. Wallop, Earl of** (1898-). British farm stock. **1950.** London: Collins. 49 pp. §
    Origins of British stock; many illustrations.
1192. **POULLE-DRIEUX, Yvonne; DUREAU-LAPEYSSONNIE, Jeanne Marie.** L'Hippiatrie dans l'occident Latin, du XII au XV siecle. **1966.** Geneve: Droz; Paris: Minard. 167 pp. §
    A bibliography of early veterinary works, with extracts of some translated into French.
1193. **POYNTER, F(rederick) N(oel) L(awrence)** (1908-). A bibliography of Gervase Markham, 1568?-1637. **1962.** Oxford: Oxford Bibliog Soc. 218 pp.
    With analysis of works on horses and vet med.
1194. **PRATT, O.S.** The horse's friend...method of educating the horse...valuable recipes, instructions in farriery... **1876.** Buffalo: The author. 536 pp.
    By self-styled professor of equine medicine.

1195. **PRICE, Willet J.** (1902-1972). Boots and forceps...as told to Hazel Heckman. **1972.** Ames, IA: Iowa State Univ. 181 pp. §
   A narrative of 40 years' pioneer vet practice.

1196. **PRINCE, Leslie B.** The farrier and his craft: the history of the Worshipful Company of Farriers. **1980.** London; New York: J.A. Allen. 260 pp.
   Includes details of blacksmithing and shoeing.

1197. **(PUBLIC HEALTH).** Veterinary medical science and human health. Senate report. **1961.** Washington: GPO. 250 pp. §
   Veterinary activities of governmental agencies.

1198. **PUGH, John.** A treatise on the science of muscular action. **1971?.** New York: Editions Medicina Rara, Facsimile 1794 ed, 106 pp. §
   With numerous finely detailed plates.

1199. **PUGH, Leslie Penrhys.** From farriery to veterinary medicine, 1785-1795. **1962.** Cambridge: RCVS. 178 pp.
   Founding and early days of the London school.

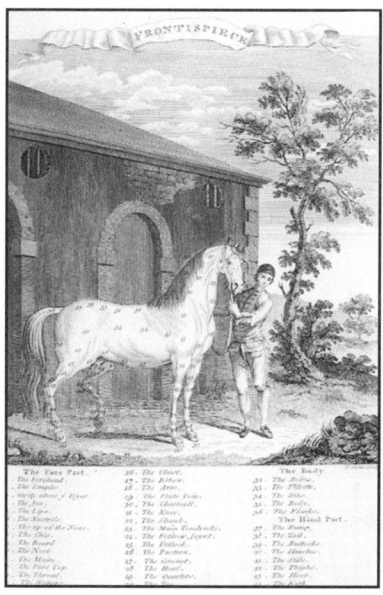

Pye: The sportsman's dictionary, 1807
(1200)

1200. **PYE, Henry James** (1745-1813). The sportsman's dictionary: containing...methods to be observed in riding...farriery, hawking, breeding and feeding horses... **1807.** London: J. Stockdale. 547 pp.
   A mediocre work including equine diseases.

1201. **QUITMAN, Edwin Leopold** (1870-). Notes on veterinary materia medica. Veterinary medicines and their uses. **1898.** Chicago: A. Eger. 202 pp. §
   A synopsis of the author's lectures.

1202.__Synopsis of Prof. Quitman's lectures on veterinary materia medica... **1903.** Chicago: A. Eger. 200 pp.

1203.__Synopsis of veterinary materia medica, therapeutics and toxicology. **1905.** Chicago: A. Eger. 2nd ed, 277 pp.

1204.__(same) **1907.** 278 pp.

1205.__(same) **1909.** 3rd ed, 278 pp.

1206.__(same) **1915.** 278 pp.

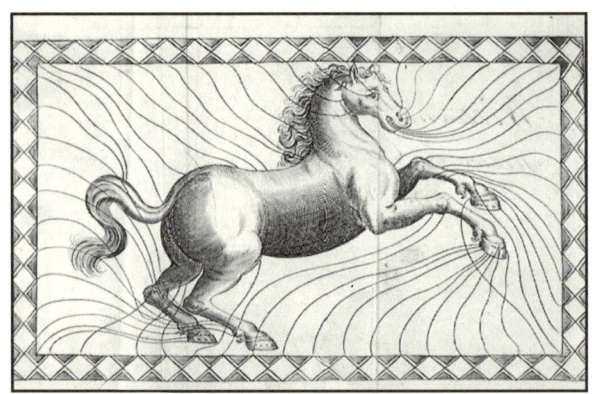

R., E.: The experienc'd farrier, 1720 (1207)

1207. **R., E.** The experienc'd farrier, or, farring compleated: containing every thing that belongs to a compleat horseman, groom, farrier or horseleach... **1720.** London: G. Conyers. 499 pp.

  A mediocre compilation; poor on diseases.

1208. **RANDALL, Henry Stephens** (1811-1876). Fine wool sheep husbandry... **1863.** New York: C.M. Saxton. 189 pp.

  A common-sense work on breeding and management.

1209.__The practical shepherd: a complete treatise on the breeding, management and diseases of sheep. **1863.** New York: Amer News Co. 452 pp.

  A useful work by an experienced sheepman.

1210.__(same) **1864.** Rochester, NY; D.D.T. Moore; Phila: J.B. Lippincott. 14th ed, 439 pp. §

1211.__Sheep husbandry...management, breeding, and the treatment of diseases. **1854.** New York: C.M. Saxton. 320 pp.

  Bound with Wm Youatt: Sheep (1848, qv).

1212. **RAREY, Caleb H.** The American art of subduing wild and vicious horses. **1860?** 7 pp.

  A brief version of J.S. Rarey's method.

1213. **RAREY, J(ohn) S(olomon)** (1827-1866). The modern art of taming wild horses. **1858.** London: G. Routledge. 63 pp. §

  Reprinted from the American edition (qv).

1214.__(same) **1856.** Columbus, OH: Ohio State Journal Co. 62 pp.

1215.__Taming, or breaking the horse: by a new and improved method...also, the complete farrier, or horse doctor... **1858?** New York: Dick & Fitzgerald. 64 pp. §

Widely reprinted work of famous American horse tamer; with mediocre farriery from Knowlson.

1216. **RAW, Nathan** (1866-). The control of bovine tuberculosis in man. **1937.** London: Bailliere, Tindall. 128 pp.

1217. **REEKS, H(arry) Caulton.** The common colics of the horse: their causes, symptoms, diagnosis, and treatment. **1902.** Chicago: A. Eger. 224 pp. §

A long-standard work, with many references.

1218.__(same) **1907.** 224 pp. §
1219.__(same) **1914.** 3rd ed, 369 pp.
1220.__(same) **1927.** London: Bailliere, Tindall. 4th ed, 403 pp. §
1221.__Diseases of the horse's foot. **1906.** Chicago: A. Eger. 458 pp. §

An excellent work advocating rational treatment.

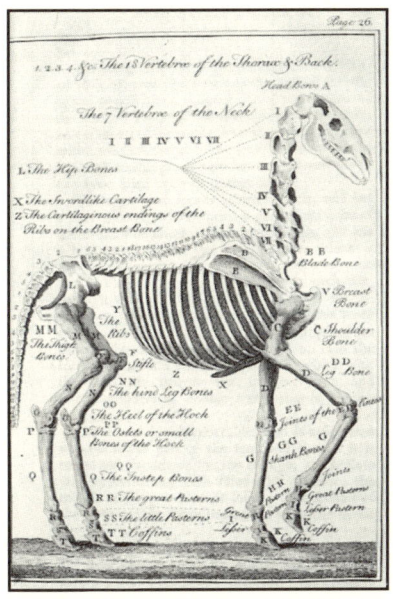

Reeves: The art of farriery, 1758 (1222)

1222. **REEVES, John.** The art of farriery both in theory and practice: containing the causes, symptoms, and cure of all diseases incident to horses... **1758.** London: J. Newbery. 478 pp. §

A better-than-average work by a farrier.

1223.__(same) **1771.** London: Carnan & Newbery. 416 pp.
1224. **REYNOLDS, Myron Herbert** (1865-). Veterinary studies for agricultural students. **1910.** New York: Macmillan. 7th ed, 290 pp. §

Generally sensible work by a noted veterinarian.

1225. **RICH, George E.** (1847-). Artistic horse-shoeing...with special directions for shaping shoes to cure different diseases of the foot... **1887.** New York: M.T. Richardson. 150 pp.
   Includes correction of faulty gaits.
1226. **RICHARDSON, Captain.** Horsemanship, or, the art of riding and managing a horse...with instructions for breaking colts and young horses. **1853.** London: Longman, Brown. 138 pp. §
   Includes buying of horses; nicely illustrated.
1227. **RICHARDSON, H.D.** Horses: their varieties, breeding, and management in health and disease. **1852.** New York: C.M. Saxton. 72 pp. §
   Sections on husbandry based largely on Youatt.
1228. **RICHARDSON, M.T.** Practical blacksmithing. **1889-90.** New York: The author. 3 vol, 232; 259; 307 pp. §
   How to set up and operate a blacksmith's shop.
1229. **RICKETTS, P.E.** The racehorse: conformation and action. **1927.** London: Constable. 54 pp.
1230. **RILEY, Harvey.** The mule. A treatise on the breeding, training, and uses, to which he may be put. **1867.** New York: Dick & Fitzgerald. 107 pp. §
   Mule husbandry, with plates of army mules in use.
1231. **RIORDAN, John J(oseph)** (1892-). Horses, mules, and remounts: the memoirs of a World War I veterinary officer. Edited by his son, John F. Riordan. **1983.** Glendale, CA: J.F. Riordan. 115 pp.
   One of few such accounts; many photographs.
1232. **ROBERGE, David.** The foot of the horse: or, lameness and all diseases of the feet traced to an unbalanced foot... **1894.** New York: W.R. Jenkins. 269 pp. §
   A rambling discourse promoting the author's idea.
1233. **ROBERTS, David** (fl 1906-1935). Dr. David Roberts' practical home veterinarian. **1910.** Waukesha, WI: The author. 10th ed, 182 pp. §
   A mediocre work promoting the author's remedies.
1234. __(same) **1912.** 10th ed, 182 pp. §
1235. __(same) **1912.** 11th ed, 184 pp. §
1236. __(same) **1930.** 20th ed, 128 pp. §
1237. **ROBERTSON, William.** A text-book of the practice of equine medicine. **1890.** London: Bailliere, Tindall. 2nd ed, 774 pp.
   Indicates good practice level at London school.
1238. **ROBINS, B.M.** Farmer's hand book or stock doctor...treatment of...horses, cattle and hogs. **1887.** Des Moines: Journal Printing. 814 pp. §
   A "cheap reliable work," generally sensible.
1239. **ROCKWELL, Andrew H.** The improved practical system of educating the horse...with an account of diseases and their treatment... **1868.** New York: Fisher & Field. 200 pp. §
   A catch-all on training, shoeing, diseases, etc.
1240. __(same) **1871.** 224 pp. §
1241. __(same) **1872.** New York: F.B. Fisher. 224 pp. §
   Includes training of cattle and dogs.

1242.__A new system of training horses: by which the wildest colts and most vicious horses can be thoroughly and safely shod... **1863**. Pierce & Budlong. 63 pp. §
   Includes the usual section on remedies.
1243. **ROE, A.H.** Horse owner's guide, being a synopsis of the diseases of horses and cattle, and how to treat them... **1878**. Elkhart, IN: Mennonite Publ Co. 128 pp. §
   Of doubtful utility; includes anatomy by Dadd.
1244. **ROE, Frank G.** The Indian and the horse. **1955**. Norman: Univ Oklahoma Press. 434 pp. §
   Some references to diseases and treatment.
1245. **ROGET, Peter Mark** (1779-1869). Animal and vegetable physiology considered with reference to natural theology. **1834**. London: W. Pickering. 2 vol, 593; 661 pp. §
   An introduction to study of natural history.
1246.__(same) **1840**. 3rd ed, 524; 598 pp.
1247. **ROHLWES, Johann Niclaus** (1755-1823). Der Taschen-Pferdearzt: ein Handbuch fur all stande, vorzuglich zum gebrauch der Kavallerie. **1810**. Berlin: F. Maurer. 316 pp. §
   A pocket manual on equine diseases.
1248.__Volstandiges Gauls-Doctor-Buch...wie der bauer und jeder Pferde-besitzer alle Krankheiten einer Pferde erkennen... **1817**. Reading, PA: H.B. Sage. 108 pp. §
   A Penna-German work on diseases of horses, etc.
1249. **ROLL, F.M.** Manuel de pathologie et therapeutique des animaux domestiques. Trans from German. **1869**. Paris: P. Asselin. 3rd ed, 2 vol, 522; 513 pp. §
   On general and special veterinary pathology.
1250. **ROPER, William.** The horse in health and disease...with instructions for stabling, training, etc. **1850?** London: F.W. Calder. 2nd ed, 117 pp. §
   Contains little useful information.
1251. **ROSEN, George.** A history of public health. **1958**. New York: MD Publications. 551 pp. §
   Includes several common animal diseases.
1252. **ROLANDSON, Thomas** (1756-1827). Medical caricatures. **1971**. New York: Editions Medicina Rara. §
   A series of 12 folio color plates.
1253. **ROWLIN, Joshua.** The complete cow-doctor, or, farmer's companion: treating of the most common disorders of black-cattle—their causes, symptoms and cures. **1794**. Glasgow: D. Niven. 275 pp.
   Mediocre, but with description of stomach tube.
1254. **RUEFF, Jakob** (1500-1558). De conceptu et generatione hominis: de matrice et eius partibus...de partu & parturientum... **1971?** New York: Editions Medicina Rara. Facsimile 1587 ed, 92 pp. §
   Facsimile of an early work on human obstetrics.

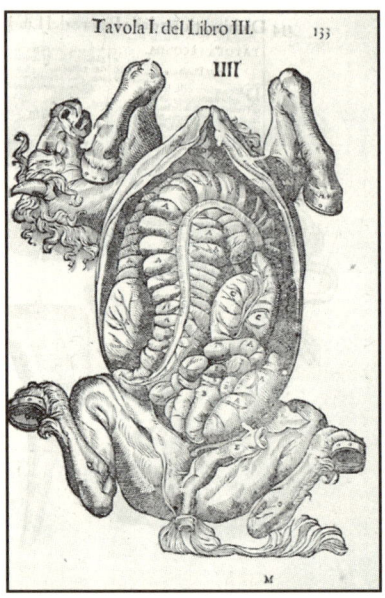

Ruini: Anatomia del cavallo, 1707 (1255)

1255. **RUINI, Carlo** (-1598). Anatomia del cavallo, infermita, et suoi rimedii... **1707**. Venetia: Lorenzo Basegio. 2 vol in 1, 250; 266 pp. §

A later edition of the classic first scientific equine anatomy (1598), with wood-block plates.

1256. **RUNNELLS, Russell A.** A guide to the study of special veterinary pathology. **1935**. Ames, IA: Collegiate Press. 218 pp. §

Superficial, but only such work then available.

1257. **RUPP, Israel Daniel** (1803-1878). The farmer's complete farrier...varieties of...the horse...with a description of all the diseases to which he is liable... **1844**. Lancaster, PA: I.L. Eshleman. 416 pp. §

A mediocre work compiled from numerous sources.

1258. **RUSH, Benjamin** (1746-1813). Medical inquiries and observations. **1809**. Phila: B. & T. Kite. 3rd ed, vol 3 (of 4). 433 pp.

Generalities on fever; details of bilious fever.

1259. __Sixteen introductory lectures. **1977**. Oceanside, NY: Dabor Science Publ. 395 pp. §

Includes lecture on diseases of animals and need for a veterinary school in America (1807).

1260. **RUSH, John.** The hand-book to veterinary homoeopathy, or, the homoeopathic treatment of the horse, the ox, the sheep, the dog and swine. **1854**. Phila: Rademacher & Sheek; New York: W. Radde. 144 pp. §

From London ed, with additions from Gunther.

1261.___(same). **1872.** New York: Boericke & Tafel. 144 pp. §
1262.___(same). **1885.** Phila: Boericke & Tafel. 144 pp. §
1263. **RUSHWORTH, William Arthur.** Sheep and their diseases. **1902.** Chicago: A. Eger. 2nd ed, 409 pp.
   For veterinary students and sheep owners.

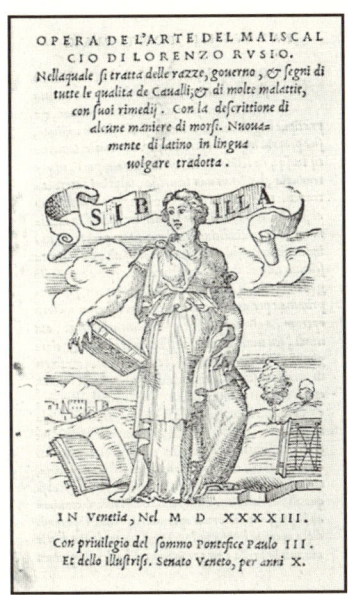

Rusius: 1543 (1264)

1264. **RUSIUS, Laurentius** (1288-1347). Opera de l'arte del malscalcio...delle razze, governo, &...le qualita de cavalli di molte malattie, con suoi remedii... **1543.** Venetia: [s.n.] 120 pp.
   Largely from other writers, but had important role in regeneration of the veterinary art.
1265. **RUSSELL, William** (1825-). Russell on scientific horseshoeing for the different diseases of the foot. **1879.** Cincinnati: R. Clarke. 142 pp. §
   A rational system, by an experienced farrier.
1266.___Russell on scientific horseshoeing for leveling and balancing the action and gait of horses and...diseases of the foot. **1901.** Cincinnati: R. Clarke. 4th ed, 295 pp.
   Rev ed, with many illustrations, some in color.
1267.___(same). **1901.** 5th ed, 315 pp.

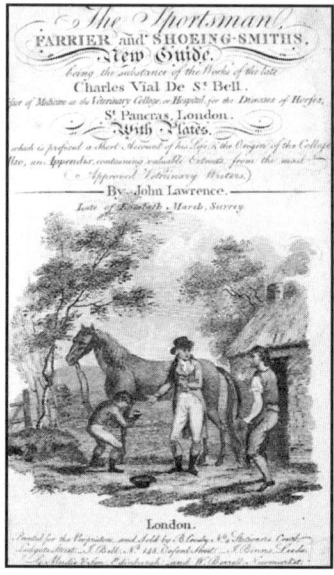

Sainbel: ca. 1800 (1269)

1268. **SAINBEL, Charles Vial de** (1753-1793). Elements of the veterinary art: containing an essay on the proportions of Eclipse...the elements of farriery...the grease, and...glanders... **1797.** London: J. Wright. 3rd ed, 127 pp. §

By the first head of the London school, whose advanced views were disregarded after he died.

1269.__The sportsman, farrier and shoeing-smiths new guide. **1800?** London: B. Crosby. 232 pp. §

A low-priced condensation of his "Elements" as compiled by John Lawrence.

1270. **SALMON, Daniel Elmer** (1850-1914). The diseases of poultry. **1899.** Washington, DC: G.E. Howard. 248 pp. §

For owners, by first chief of USDA BAI.

1271.__(same). **1899.** Washington, DC: Feather Publ Co. 248 pp.

1272. **SAMPLE, H.** The horse and dog: not as they are, but as they should be...together with an essay on horseshoeing. **1882.** San Francisco: [s.n.]. 280 pp. §

Mainly on the horse, including diseases.

1273. **SANDERS, James Harvey** (1832-1899). Horse-breeding: being the general principles of heredity applied to the business of breeding horses... **1893.** Chicago: The author. 428 pp.

A guide to breeding stud management.

1274. **SAUNDERS, Charles G(reatley)** (1875-). Canine medicine and surgery. **1915.** Chicago: Amer Jnl Vet Med. 249 pp. §

A basic work for students and practitioners.

1275. **SAUNDERS, C.** Rabbit and cat diseases. **1920.** Chicago: Amer Vet Publ. 121 pp.

A practical work for owners.

1276. **SAUNDERS, L(eon) Z.** (1919-). Veterinary pathology in Russia, 1860-1930. **1980.** Ithaca, NY: Cornell Univ Press. 327 pp. §
Details of formerly obscure scientists, etc.

1277. **SAUNDERS, Simon W.** Domestic poultry... **1867.** New York: O. Judd. 120 pp. §
Written for neophytes and fanciers.

1278. **SAVAGE, William G(eorge)** (1872-1961). The prevention of tuberculosis of bovine origin. **1929.** London: Macmillan. 195 pp.
Prevalence of TB and methods of control.

1279. **SCHAEFER, J.C.** New manual of homoeopathic veterinary medicine...adapted to the use of every owner of domestic animals... **1871.** New York; San Francisco: Boericke & Tafel. 312 pp. §
Includes directions for drug preparation.

1280. __(same). **1873.** New York; San Francisco: Boericke & Tafel; Phila: F.E. Boericke. 321 pp. §

1281. __(same). **1880.** New York: Boericke & Tafel. 321 pp. §

1282. **SCHALK, Arthur Frederick** (1880-). History of the College of Veterinary Medicine, The Ohio State University 1873-1956. **1957.** Columbus: OSU Press. 116 pp. §
With lists of faculty and graduates.

1283. **SCHALLER, Oskar; POBISCH, Richard** (eds). Bericht uber die 200-Jahr-Feier der Tierarztlichen Hochschule in Wien. **1970.** Wien: Tierarzt Hochschule. 181 pp.
Bicentennary volume of the Vienna school.

1284. **SCHAUDER, W.** Zur Geschicte der Veterinar-Medizin an der Universitat und Justus Liebig-Hochschule. **1957?** [s.l. s.n.] 178 pp. §
A history of the Giessen school, 1607-1957.

1285. **SCHMIDT, Hubert** (1886-1958). Eighty years of veterinary medicine at the Agricultural and Mechanical College of Texas... 1878-1958. **1958.** College Station, TX: College Archives. 40 pp. §
With numerous early photographs.

1286. **SCHNELLE, Gerry B.** Radiology in canine practice A text on applied radiography and diagnosis. **1945.** Evanston, IL: No Amer Vet. 336 pp. §
The first text of its kind in English.

1287. **SCHUH, Herman Loy.** The practice of veterinary surgery...lectures delivered to the seniors of the Grand Rapids Veterinary College. **1912.** Grand Rapids, MI: The College. 260 pp. §

1288. **SCHULTZ, James A.** (1836-). The horse and its diseases: embracing a list of medicines used generally used in horse practice, and their properties... **1879.** Middletown, NY: Stivers & Slauson. 95 pp. §
Much miscellaneous material; author signature.

1289. **SCHWABE, Calvin W.** Cattle, priests, and progress in medicine. **1978.** Minneapolis: Univ Minn Press. 277 pp.
Vet medicine and advances in human medicine.

1290.___Veterinary medicine and human health. **1984.** Baltimore: Williams & Wilkins. 3rd ed, 680 pp.

A historical approach to the interface between human and veterinary medicine.

1291.___; **RIEMANN, Hans; FRANTI, Charles E.** Epidemiology in veterinary practice. **1977.** Phila: Lea & Febiger. 303 pp.

Extensive bibliographies with historical items.

1292. **SCOFIELD, Samuel.** A practical treatise on vaccinia, or cow pock. **1810.** New York: Collins & Perkins. 139 pp.

Prevention and treatment of pox in man.

1293. **SCUDDER, Charles Locke** (1860-). The treatment of fractures, with notes upon a few common dislocations. **1907.** Phila; London: W.B. Saunders. 6th ed, 628 pp.

A basic human text.

1294. **SCULTETUS, Johannes** (1595-1645). Cheiroplotheke ...armamentarium chirurgicum XLIII...medicinae pariter ac chirugiae studiosis perutile... **1971?** New York: Editions Medicina Rara. Facsimile 1655 ed, 67 pp. §

Facsimile of Ulm ed, with many plates.

1295. **SETON, Ernest Thompson** (1860-1946). Studies in the art anatomy of animals... **1896.** London; New York: Macmillan. 96 pp.

With 49 large plates of wild animals and birds.

1296. **SEUTER, Mang.** Ein vast schones und nutzliches Beuch von der Rossartzney...zu dem auch von vilen guetten und erfarnen Hueffschmiden zu wegen... **1588.** Augspurg: M. Manger. 440 pp.

A major 16thC work on equine diseases.

1297. **SEWELL, Louis.** Canine distemper, a practical handbook. **1925.** London: G. Routledge. 218 pp.

An early work on a major disease problem.

1298. **SHARE-JONES, John T.** The surgical anatomy of the horse. **1907.** New York: W.R. Jenkins. 4 vol, 159; 190; 220; 259 pp.

A regional text with many plates, some in color.

1299. **SHARP, Walter N.** Ophthalmology for veterinarians. **1913.** Phila: W.B. Saunders. 210 pp. §

A concise textbook, primarily for students.

1300. **SHOSHAN, A.** Animals in Jewish literature. **1971.** Rehovot, Israel: The author. 124 + 372 pp. §

A series of articles in English and Hebrew.

1301. **SHUMWAY, Henry L.** A hand-book on tuberculosis among cattle, with considerations of the relation of the disease to the health and life of the human family, and...use of tuberculin as a diagnostic test. **1895.** Boston: Roberts Bros. 178 pp. §

Written by a journalist to inform the public.

1302. **SIEDAMGROTZKH, D.** (compiler). Die Veterinarpolizei-Gesetze und Verordnungen fur...Thierarzte und Landwirthe. **1881.** Dresden: Schonfeld. 198 pp.
State veterinary hygiene in Germany.

1303. **SIME, D.** Rabies. **1903.** Cambridge: Cambridge Univ Press. 290 pp. §
The rabies virus and methods of transmission.

1304. **SIMMONDS, Peter Lund** (1814-1897). Animal products: their preparation, commercial uses and value. **1889.** London: Chapman & Hall. 416 pp.
Uses of products from domestic and wild animals.

1305. **SIMMONS, John** (compiler). The American farrier...diseases incident to horses, and prescriptions for their cure... **1825.** Phila: The compiler. 144 pp. §
Somewhat better than most works of this genre.

1306. **SIMONDS, James Beart** (1810-1904). A practical treatise on variola ovina, or small-pox in sheep...with the progress, symptoms, and treatment of the disease... **1848.** London: J. Ridgway. 157 pp. §
A detailed work with color plates.

1307. **SIMPSON, George G.** Horses: the story of the horse family...through sixty million years of history. **1951.** New York: Oxford Univ Press. 247 pp. §
The fossil record and evolution of the horse.

1308. **SINCLAIR, Upton.** The jungle. **1980.** New York: New American Library. 350 pp. §
An expose (c 1905) of the meat-packing industry that resulted in USDA meat inspection system.

1309. **SIND, J.B. von** (1709?-1776). L'art du manege pris dans ses vrais principes...pour l'embouchure des chevaux et...des principales maladies... **1773.** Berlin: C.F. Himbourg. 317 pp.
On equitation and diseases of the horse.

1310.__Vollstandiger unterricht in den Wissenschaften eines Stallmeisters. **1770.** Gottingen: J.C. Dieterich. 324 pp. §
A classic on equine management and diseases.

1311.__(same) **1775.** 1314 pp. §

1312. **SISSON, Septimus** (1865-1924). The anatomy of the domestic animals. **1914.** Phila; London: W.B. Saunders. 930 pp. §
A standard text for 50+ years.

1313.__(same) **1917.** 2nd ed, 930 pp. §

1314.__(same) **1930.** 930 pp. §

1315.__Ligaments and muscles of the horse. **1895.** Toronto: J.A. Carveth. 56 pp. §
The principal structures in outline form.

1316.__A text-book of veterinary anatomy. **1910.** Phila; London: W.B. Saunders. 826 pp. §
Forerunner of item 1312.

1317. **SKEAVINGTON, George.** The horse and veterinary practice described and illustrated, in the management of horses, dogs, cattle, sheep, pigs, poultry, etc... **1850.** London: London Printing. 1016 pp.
Compiled from various sources, including Youatt.

96 *Five Centuries of Veterinary Medicine*

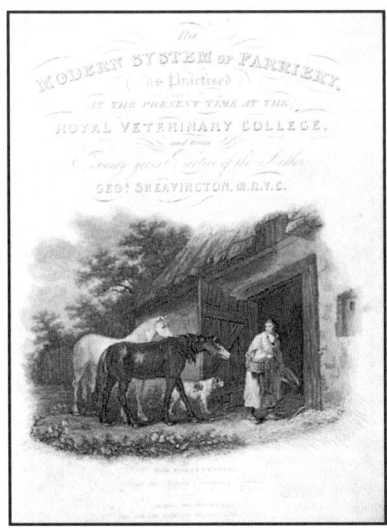

Skeavington: ca. 1850 (1318)

1318.__The modern system of farriery: comprehending the...mode of practice...at the Royal Veterinary College... **1850?** London; New York: London Printing. 523 pp.
A work for horse owners, with large plates.

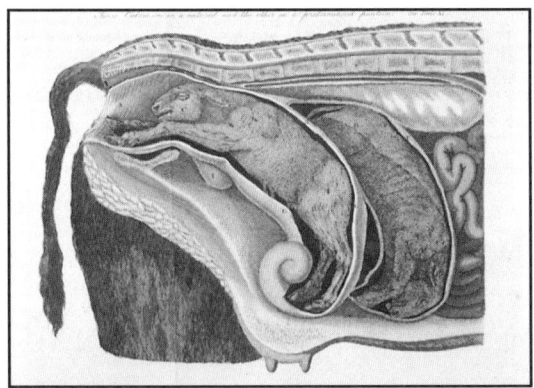

Skellett: A practical treatise on the breeding cow, 1807
(1319)

1319. **SKELLETT, Edward.** A practical treatise on the breeding cow and extraction of the calf...in which the question of difficult parturition is considered... **1807.** London: Sherwood, Gilbert. 364 pp.
A superb work, with large plates in color.
1320.__A practical treatise on the parturition of the cow...and on the diseases of neat cattle in general... **1822.** London: Sherwood, Neely. 364 pp.
Essentially like the 1807 edition.

1321. **SLOAN, Walter B.** The complete farrier or horse doctor: also, the complete cattle doctor... **1849.** Chicago: The author. 3rd ed, 160 pp.
  A mediocre work promoting Sloan's remedies.
1322.__(same) **1851.** 4th ed, 160 pp.
1323.__Sloan's complete farrier and cattle doctor...with a full account of all the diseases... **1869.** Chicago: Walker & Taylor. 5th ed, 319 pp. §
  A greatly enlarged but little improved edition.
1324. **SMITH, Andrew** (-1914). Veterinary notes...on the causes, symptoms and treatment of the diseases of domestic animals... **1885.** Toronto: J.A. Carveth. 252 pp.
  By founder (1862) of Ontario Veterinary College.
1325.__(same) **1889.** Rev ed, 225 pp.
1326.__(same) **1891.** 225 pp. §
1327. **SMITH, Arthur Croxton** (1865-). British dogs. **1945.** London: Collins. 47 pp. §
  A brief history, nicely illustrated.

Sir Frederick Smith (1857-1929)

1328.__The early history of veterinary literature and its British development. **1976.** London: J.A. Allen. 4 vol, 373; 244; 184; 161 pp. (Reprint)
  Vol 1. Earliest times to 1700; vol 2. 18thC; vol 3. 1800-1823; vol 4. 1824-1866.
1329.__(same) Vol 2. **1924;** vol 3. **1930;** vol 4. **1933.** London: Bailliere, Tindall. §
  Vol 1 ran in J Comp Path Therap 26-30: 1913-17.
1330.__A history of the Royal Army Veterinary Corps, 1796-1929. **1927.** London: Bailliere, Tindall. 268 pp.
  Includes chapter on the army farrier 1600-1796.
1331.__A manual of veterinary hygiene. **1905.** London: Bailliere, Tindall. 5th ed, 1035 pp. §
  Includes government regs and military hygiene.
1332.__(same) **1906.** New York: W.R. Jenkins. 5th ed, 1035 pp.
1333.__A manual of veterinary physiology. **1892.** London: Bailliere, Tindall. 401 pp. §
  An early text on the subject, widely used.
1334.__(same) **1900.** New York: W.R. Jenkins. 2nd ed, 573 pp.
1335.__(same) **1903.** 573 pp.
1336.__(same) **1904.** 573 pp.
1337.__(same) **1906.** 503 pp.
1338.__(same) **1912.** Chicago: A. Eger. 4th ed, 808 pp. §
  With addition of clinical aspects and a large section on generation and development.
1339.__(same) **1912.** London: Bailliere, Tindall. 808 pp. §

1340. **SMITH, Howard Remus** (1872-). The conquest of bovine tuberculosis in the United States. **1959.** Somerset, MI: The author. 2nd ed. 63 pp. §
　Vignettes of early days of TB eradication.
1341. **SMITH, H.R. Bradley.** Blacksmith and farriers tools at Shelburne Museum. **1966.** Shelburne, VT: The museum. 271 pp. §
　A detailed history, including that of nails.
1342. **SMITH, Robert Meade** (1854-). The physiology of the domestic animals: a text-book for veterinary and medical students and practitioners. **1890.** Phila; London: F.A. Davis. 938 pp. §
　By a physician; probably considered academic at the time; J.V. Lacroix signature.
1343.__(same) **1907.** Chicago: A. Eger. 938 pp.
1344. **SMITHCORS, J(ames) F(rederick)** (1920-). The American veterinary profession, its background and development. **1963.** Ames, IA: ISU Press. 704 pp. §
　From colonial times to AVMA centennial (1963); signed by author.
1345.__Evolution of the veterinary art: a narrative account to 1850. **1957.** Kansas City, MO: Vet Med Publ Co. 408 pp. §
　From earliest times to 18thC Britain (excludes United States); signed by author.
1346.__The first 100 years: history of the AVMA 1863-1963. **1959-63.** Chicago: Amer Vet Med Assn. (photocopy) 105 pp. §
　A series of 100 articles appearing in JAVMA in connection with the AVMA centennial (1963).
1347.__The veterinarian in America, 1625-1975. **1975.** Santa Barbara, CA: Amer Vet Publ. 160 pp. §
　A copiously illustrated, large-format work.
1348. **SMYTHE, Reginald Harrison.** Healers on horseback: the reminiscences of an English veterinary surgeon. **1963.** Springfield, IL: C. C Thomas. 135 pp. §
　Anecdotes of early 20thC British practice.

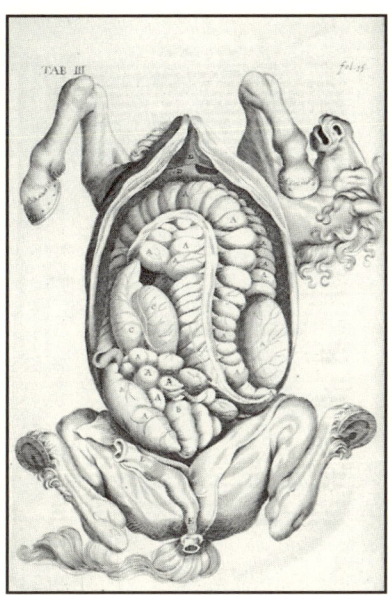

Snape: The anatomy of an horse, 1683
(1349)

1349. **SNAPE, Andrew** (1644-). The anatomy of an horse: containing an exact and full description of the frame, situation and connexion of all his parts. **1683.** London: The author. 237 pp + 45-p appendix.

The first equine anatomy in English, with plates based on Ruini but reversed, and appendix on circulation and generation based on Harvey.

1350. **SNYDER, William.** Hand-book to veterinary medicine, or, a treatise on the sick horse... **1870.** Adrian, MI: Times & Expositor. 16 pp. §

Mediocre; "for those lacking larger works."

1351. **SOLLEYSEL, Jacques de** (1617-1680). The compleat horseman, or, perfect farrier...Part I discovering the surest marks of the beauty...and perfections of horses...Part II contains the signs and causes of their diseases... **1702.** London: H. Bonwicke. 376 pp. §

An abridgment of the Hope trans (of item 1353) which brought Solleysel's views to Britain.

1352.__(same) **1711.** London: R. Bonwicke, W. Freeman. 2nd ed, 376 pp.

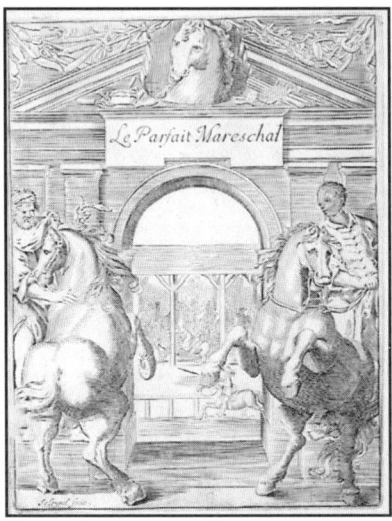

Solleysel: 1682 (1353)

1353.___Le parfait mareschal, qui enseigne a connoistre la beaute, la bonte, et la deffauts des chevaux ; les signes...des maladies... **1682**. Paris: G. Clouzier. 5th ed, 2 vol in 1, 556; 410 pp. §

A classic work by an enlightened practitioner responsible for reformation of French practice.

1354.___(same) **1691**. A la Haye: H. Van Bulderen. 8th ed, 2 vol, 250; 398 pp. §

1355. **SOMMERFELD, Paul.** Methods for the examination of milk: for chemists, physicians and hygienists. **1901**. Chicago: A. Eger. 96 pp. §

Chemical and physical properties of milk.

1356. **SOMERVILLE, William** (1675-1742). The chace. A poem. **1735**. London: G. Hawkins. 106 pp. §

A classic; includes dog diseases, esp rabies. Bound with: Hobbinol, or the rural games. **1740**.

1357. **(SPAIN).** Secunda asamblea nacional veterinaria, celebrada en Madrid... **1907**. Madrid: R. Alvarez. 377 pp.

Papers presented at Natl Vet Assn meeting.

1358. **SPAULDING, Roy H(enry)** (1893-). Your dog and your cat...a treatise on the care... **1921**. New York; London: D. Appleton. 166 pp.

A largely sensible book for owners.

1359. **SPOONER, William Charles** (1809?-1885). Appendix to the horse, as published by the Society for the Diffusion of Useful Knowledge... **1850**. London: Robert Baldwin. 192 pp. §

Various topics keyed to Youatt: The horse (qv).

1360.___A treatise on the structure, functions, and diseases of the foot and leg of the horse...the subject of shoeing and the proper treatment of the foot... **1840**. London: Longman, Orme. 337 pp. §

A well-written sensible work.

1361.__Veterinary art: a practical treatise on the diseases of the horse. **1851.** London: J.J. Griffen. 2nd ed, 107 pp.
    Appeared in Encyclopaedia Metropolitana (1848).
ST BEL, Charles Vial de—see Sainbel, Vial de.
1362. **STALHEIM, Ole H.V.** (ed). Veterinary medicine in the west. **1988.** Manhattan, KS: Sunflower Univ Press. 266 pp.
    A series of articles by 12 veterinarians.
1363. **STANGE, C(harles H(enry)** (1880-1936). History of veterinary medicine at Iowa State College... 1879-1929. **1929.** Ames, IA: [s.n.] 96 pp. §
    With numerous biographies and early photos.
1364. **STEEL, John Henry.** A treatise on the diseases of the dog: being a manual of canine pathology... **1888.** London: Longmans, Green. 287 pp.
    A well-organized and useful work.
1365.__(same) **1894.** New York: Wiley. 287 pp.
1366.__A treatise on diseases of the ox: being a manual of bovine pathology... **1887.** London: Longmans, Green. 2nd ed, 520 pp. §
    Written for students and practitioners.
1367.__(same) **1887.** New York: Wiley. 520 pp.
1368.__A treatise on the diseases of the sheep: being a manual of ovine pathology... **1890.** London: Longmans, Green. 362 pp.
    A first-rate work; includes section on poisons.
1369. **STEFFEN, Mart(in) R(obert)** (1882) The clinical diagnosis of cattle diseases. **1917.** Detroit: Detroit Vet Supply. 127 pp. §
    A superficial discussion of common diseases.
1370.__Special cattle therapy. **1915.** Chicago: Amer Jnl Vet Med. 157 pp. §
    A practical work based on experience.
1371.__Special equine therapy. **1917.** Chicago: Amer Jnl Vet Med. 212 pp. §
    Briefly covers treatment of common diseases.
1372.__Special veterinary therapy. **1914.** Chicago: Amer Jnl Vet Med. 97 pp. §
    Superficial coverage of various topics.
1373.__A treatise on regional iodine therapy for the veterinary clinician. **1919.** New York: Pharmacal Advance Publ Co. 63 pp. §
    Antisepsis and treatment of skin diseases.
1374.__Veterinary clinical notes. **1917.** Brillon, WI: Chemic-Specialty Co. 180 pp. §
    Practical observations on diagnosis and therapy. Second copy with E.A. Ehmer signature.
1375. **(STEPHEN, George, Sir)** (1794-1879) (pseud Caveat Emptor). The adventures of a gentleman in search of a horse. **1836.** London: Saunders & Otley. 2nd ed, 376 pp.
    Advice to purchasers, with legal citations.
1376.__(same) **1836.** Phila: Carey, Lea. 288 pp. §
1377. **STEPHENS, Henry** (1795-1874). The book of the farm: detailing the labors of the farmer, steward...cattle-man, shepherd...and dairymaid. **1860.** New York: C.M. Saxton. Vol 2, 462 pp. §
    Includes parturition of cows, ewes and mares.

1378. **STEWART, Henry.** The shepherd's manual. A practical treatise on the sheep... **1876.** New York: O. Judd. 752 pp. §
   Includes a mediocre short section on diseases.
1379. **STEWART, John.** Stable economy: a treatise on the management of horses... **1838.** Edinburgh: W. Blackwood; London: T. Cadell. 432 pp.
   Advises calling veterinarian for diseases.
1380.__(same) **1840.** 3rd ed, 436 pp. §
1381.__(same) **1845.** New York: D. Appleton; Phila: G.S. Appleton. 378 pp. §
1382. **STEWART, R.W.** Veterinary notes. **1887?** [s.l. s.n.] 237 pp.
   Identical to Smith: Veterinary notes (1885).
1383. **STEWART, Robert.** The American farmer's horse book: embracing...the several diseases peculiar to the American horse...together with...modes of treatment... **1867.** Richmond; Atlanta; New Orleans: Natl Publ Co. 600 pp.
   A useful work by an experienced practitioner.
1384.__(same) **1868.** Cincinnati: C.F. Vent; Chicago: J.S. Goodman. 600 pp. §
1385.__(same) **1871.** Cincinnati; New York: C.F. Vent; Chicago: J.S. Goodman. 600 pp.
1386.__Das Pferdebuch des Amerikanischen farmers: enthaltend eine ausfuhrliche beschreibung der...Pferdekrankheiten... **1866?** Milwaukee, WI G. Brunder. 592 pp. §
   German edition of Stewart's horse book.
1387. **STILES, Charles Wardell** (1867-1941). The inspection of meats for animal parasites: I. The flukes and tapeworms of cattle, sheep, and swine...II. Compendium of the parasites... **1898.** Washington: GPO. 161 pp. §
   A handbook for meat inspectors, by a zoologist.
1388.__Trichinosis in Germany. **1901.** Washington: GPO. 24 pp. §
Prevalence, with alleged case of US origin.
1389. **STILLMAN, J(acob) D(avis) B(abcock)** (1819-1888). The horse in motion as shown by instantaneous photography, with a study on animal mechanics...in which is demonstrated the theory of quadrupedal locomotion... **1882.** Boston: Osgood. 127 pp.
   The famous Muybridge plates depicting gaits.
1390. **STOCKHAM, Steven L.; BERRIER, Harry H.** History of the American Society for Veterinary Clinical Pathology: 1965-1985. **1986.** [s.l.] The Society. 78 pp.
1391. **STOCKTON, Jack J.** (ed). A century of service: veterinary medicine in Indiana, 1884-1984. **1984.** Indianapolis: Indiana VMA. 199 pp.
   With emphasis on Association matters.
   STONEHENGE—see John Henry Walsh
1392. **STORKE, Elliot G.** (1811-1879). The domestic animals: embracing I. the horse...II. cattle...III. sheep...IV. the pig...V. poultry... **1859.** Auburn, NY: Auburn Publ Co. 311 pp.
   Breeds and management, from various sources.
1393. (**STRANGEWAYS, Thomas**) (1824-1869). Strangeways' veterinary anatomy, ed by I. Vaughn. **1879.** Edinburgh: Bell & Bradfute. 2nd ed, 572 pp.
   A long-standard text in Britain and America.

1394.__(same) **1886.** Edinburgh: Bell & Bradfute; London: Simpkin, Marshall. 3rd ed, 601 pp. §

1395.__(same) **1900.** New York: W.R. Jenkins. 4th ed, 597 pp.

1396.__(same) **1901.** 597 pp. §

1397. **STROTHER, Edward** (1675-1737). The practical physician for travellers: whether by sea or land. **1729.** London: F. Fayram. 132 pp.

A do-it-yourself work for travellers.

1398. **STUART, George.** The stock breeders' manual. Breeding, rearing, and treatment of diseases of farm stock... **1888.** Cleveland: Whitworth Bros. 267 pp.

A mediocre work promoting the author's remedies.

1399. **STUBBS, E(van) L.** (1890-). A history of veterinary medicine in Pennsylvania. **1962?** [s.l. s.n.] 27 pp. §

A superficial coverage of various topics.

George Stubbs (1724-1806)

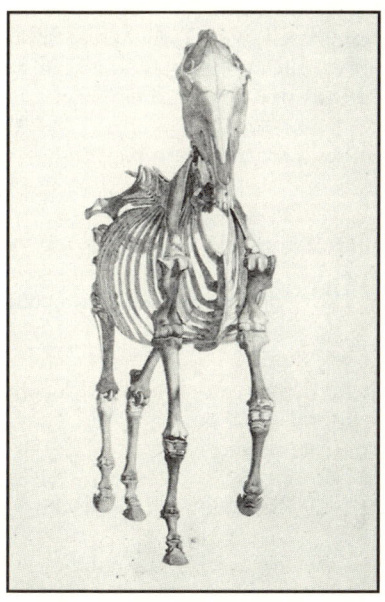

Stubbs: The anatomy of the horse, 1766
(1400)

1400.__The anatomy of the horse: including a particular description of the bones, cartilages, muscles, fascias, ligaments, nerves, arteries, veins, and glands...all done from nature. **1766.** London: The author. 47 pp, 24 leaves of plates. §

A large-folio classic by the noted animal painter; one of only 150 copies printed.

1401.(__) **McCUNN, James** (1894-). The anatomy of the horse: the original 1766 edition and illustrations, with a modern veterinary paraphrase... **1965.** London: J.A. Allen. 147 pp.
   With 24 previously unpublished plates.
1402.(__) **DOHERTY, Terence.** The anatomical works of George Stubbs. **1974.** London: Secker & Warburg. 345 pp, mainly illustrations. §
   All of Stubbs' anatomical works, animal & human.
1403.(__) **EGERTON, Judy.** George Stubbs, anatomist and animal painter. **1976.** London: Tate Gallery. 64 pp, numerous plates. §
   A biography, with several anatomical plates.
1404.(__) **GAUNT, William.** Stubbs. **1977.** Oxford: Phaidon. 16 pp text, 48 folio color plates. §
   A magnificent selection, mainly of horses, etc.
1405.(__) **HALL, William Henry.** System of farriery ... **1791.** [s.l.]: Extract from The New Royal Encyclopaedia Vol 1, 20 pp + 6 folio plates, disbound. §
   An abridgement of Stubbs' Anatomy, with a section on diseases added.
1406.(__) **SPARROW, Walter Shaw** (1862-1940). George Stubbs and Ben Marshall. **1929.** London: Cassell; New York: Scribner. 80 pp + plates. §
   A good account of the life and work of these famous animal painters.
1407.(__) **TATTERSALL, Bruce.** Stubbs and Wedgewood. **1974.** London: Tate Gallery. 119 pp. §
   An account of Stubbs' excursion into painting on enamel, reproduced on Wedgewood plaques.

1408. **SURTEES, Robert Smith** (1805-1864). Ask mama... **18—**. London: Bradbury, Agnew. 423 pp. §
   One of a series of 18thC sporting novels, with color plates by John Leech, et al.
1409.__Handley Cross... 578 pp. §
1410.__Hawbuck Grange... 265 pp. §
1411.__Mr. Romford's hounds. 423 pp. §
1412.__Mr. Sponge's sporting tour. 450 pp. §
1413.__Plain or ringlets? 406 pp. §
1414.__Young Tom Hall... **1926.** Edinburgh: W. Blackwood; New York: Scribners. 359 pp. §
   Includes chapter on dealing in crippled horses.
1415. **SUZOR, Renaud.** Hydrophobia, an account of M. Pasteur's system, containing a translation of all his communications on the subject... **1887.** London: Chatto & Windus. 231 pp.
1416. **SVINHUFVUD, Anne Charlotte** (ed). A late Middle English treatise on horses...from British Library MS. Sloane 2584, ff. 102-117b. **1978.** Stockholm: Almqvist & Wiksell. 281 pp. §
   On horsemanship, with facsimile of original.
1417. **SWANZY, Henry Rosborough, Sir** (1843-1913). A handbook of the diseases of the eye and their treatment. **1900.** Phila: P. Blakiston's Sons. 7th ed, 607 pp.
   A comprehensive human text.

1418. **TABOURIN, Francois** (1818-). Nouveau traite de matiere medicale de therapeutique et de pharmacie veterinaires... **1853.** Paris: V. Masson. 831 pp. §
   An exhaustive work based on mode of drug action.
1419.__(same) **1875.** Paris: P. Asselin. 3rd ed, 2 vol, 820; 740 pp. §
   With 16 pp catalog of veterinary books, etc.
1420. **TAGGART, John.** The horse: his diseases and treatment. **1869.** Lancaster, PA: J.M. Westhaeffer. 75 pp.
   A mediocre work with many harsh remedies.

William Taplin (1740?-1807)

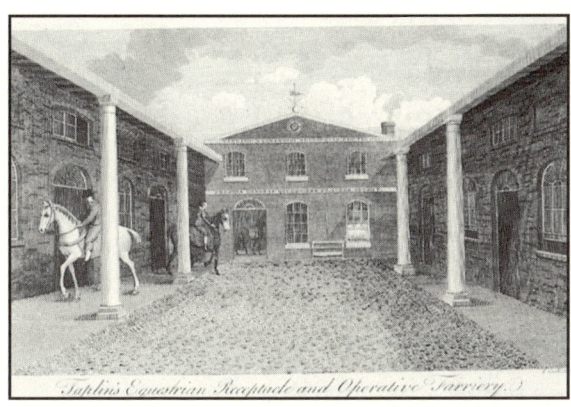

Taplin: A compendium of practical and experimental farriery, 1796 (1421)

1421.__A compendium of practical and experimental farriery...suggested by reason and confirmed by practice... **1796.** London: P. Norbury. 274 pp. §
   A condensation of the Stable directory (qv).
1422.__(same) **1797.** Wilmington, DE: Bonsal & Niles. 290 pp.
   Abridged from the English edition.
1423.__The gentleman's stable directory, or, modern system of farriery. **1788.** London: G. Kearsley. 356 pp. §
   By a surgeon ignorant of veterinary practice; full of hideous errors, repeated many times.
1424.__(same) **1791.** 419 pp. §
1425.__(same) **1796.** London: G.G. & J. Robinson. Vol 1, 13th ed, 502 pp. §
1426.__(same) **1796.** Vol 2, 4th ed, 416 pp. §
   A companion volume to preceding item.
1427.__(same) **1812.** Phila: J. Webster. Vol 1 & 2, New ed, 540 pp. §
   Essentially the same as London 1796 editions.
1428.__The sporting dictionary and rural repository of general information upon...the sports of the field. **1803.** London: Vernor & Hood. 2 vol, 526; 506 pp. §
   Includes veterinary topics of doubtful value.

1429.(__) The American farrier, or, New-York horse doctor... **1826**. Troy, NY: F. Adancourt. 188 pp. §

A rehash of Taplin by "an experienced farrier."

1430.(__) The sportsman's cabinet, or a correct delineation of the canine race. **1803-04**. London: The "proprietors" [Taplin]. 2 vol, 276; 310 pp. §

A sumptuous work with elegant plates but little worthwhile information on dog disease.

1431.(__) Taplin improved, or, a compendium of farriery: wherein is fully explained the...diseases and accidents...and the methods of cure... **1811**. London: B. Crosby. 144 pp. §

A wretched posthumous work of no redeeming value.

1432. **TELLOR, LLOYD V.** The diseases of livestock and their most efficient remedies...giving in brief and plain language a description of all the usual diseases... **1879**. Phila: H.C. Watts. 469 pp. §

A mediocre work by a neophyte; includes hornail.

1433.__(same) **1881**. Phila: H.C. Watts; Cincinnati: Forshee & McMartin. 499 pp. §

1434. **TENNECKER, Christian E.S. Ritter von** (1770-1839). Lehrbuch der Pferdearztlichen Geburtshulfe und Heiling der gewohnlichsten Krankheiten der Mutterstuten und Fohlen... **1820**. Prag: F. Tempsky. 523 pp.

An early work on equine obstetrics.

1435. **TESSIER, Alexandre Henri** (1741-1837). A complete treatise on Merinos and other sheep. **1811**. New York: Economical School Office. 175 pp. §

Translated from French; includes diseases.

1436. **THATCHER, James** (1754-1844). The American new dispensatory... medical prescriptions...medical uses of the gases...medical electricity. **1813**. Boston: Thomas B. Wait. 732 pp. §

A materia medica and pharmacopoeia.

1437.__Observations on hydrophobia, produced by the bite of a mad dog, or other rabid animal...the various theories and methods of cure... **1812**. Plymouth, MA: J. Avery. 301 pp. §

The first extensive report of rabies in America.

1438. **THOMPSON, Charles** (1710?-). Rules for bad horsemen... **1765**. London: J. Robson. 84 pp. §

Elementary axioms for neophyte riders.

1439. **THOMPSON, J.** Modern practice of farriery, or, complete horse doctor...the most approved cures for the several diseases to which horses are subject... **1807**. Phila: J. Crukshank. 152 pp. §

British reprint; remedies from earlier time.

1440. **THOMPSON, Ray** (1926-). After 1883: one hundred years of organized veterinary medicine in Pennsylvania... **1982**. Harrisburg, PA: Penna VMA/W.B. Saunders. 235 pp. §

A nicely written and elegantly illustrated work.

1441.__The feisty veterinarians of New Jersey: their first one hundred years. **1984.** Rockaway, NJ: New Jersey VMA. 254 pp. §

A highly readable person-oriented history.

1442.__The good doctors. **1986.** Fallston, MD: Maryland VMA. 246 pp. §

A 100-year history of veterinary medicine in Maryland, with many photos; signed by author.

1443. **THOMPSON, Ruth D'Arcy** (1902-). The remarkable Gamgees: a story of achievement. **1974.** Edinburgh: Ramsay Head Press. 216 pp.

A biography of the Gamgee family, by a great-granddaughter of the founding father.

1444. **THRESHER, Leonard.** The family physician, nurse's guide, and farmer's horse and cattle doctor. **1871.** Montpelier, VT: Argus & Patriot. 406 pp.

With mediocre sections on domestic animals.

1445. **TITUS, Nelson N.** The American eclectic practice of medicine, as applied to the diseases of domestic animals... **1865.** Union, NY: The author. 280 pp.

Enlightened ideas on bloodletting, hornail, etc.

1446. **TODD, Charles.** Description of the serum institute (abbassia) and of the preparation of cattle plague serum. **1912.** Cairo: Government Press. 34 pp.

1447. **TOPHAM, Thomas.** A new compendious system on several diseases incident to cattle...calves...horses. **1788.** London: J. Scatherd & J. Whitaker. 421 pp. Bound with Clater: Cattle doctor 1817 (qv).

By a physician hoping to rescue cattle from quackery; an original but uninspired work.

1448. **TOWAR, Alexander.** Der Amerikanische Pferdearzt ...so wie auch eine Beschriebung aller Krankheiten...alle Krankheiten des Rindviehs...der Schaafe... **1832.** Phila: The author. 240 pp.

A Penna-German work, from earlier German source.

1449. **TREW, Cecil G.** The horse through the ages. **1953.** London: Methuen. 75 pp. §

From prehistory through 18thC; illustrated.

1450. **TRUE, Alfred Charles** (1853-1929). A history of agricultural experimentation and research in the United States, 1607-1925: including a history of the United States Department of Agriculture. **1937.** Washington: GPO. 321 pp. §

Includes numerous references to animal disease.

1451. **TUFFNELL, F.** The gentleman's pocket-farrier: shewing how to use your horse on a journey...remedies for common accidents that may befal him on the road. **1832.** Boston: Carter & Hendee. 34 pp.

With sensible precautions against harsh methods.

108   *Five Centuries of Veterinary Medicine*

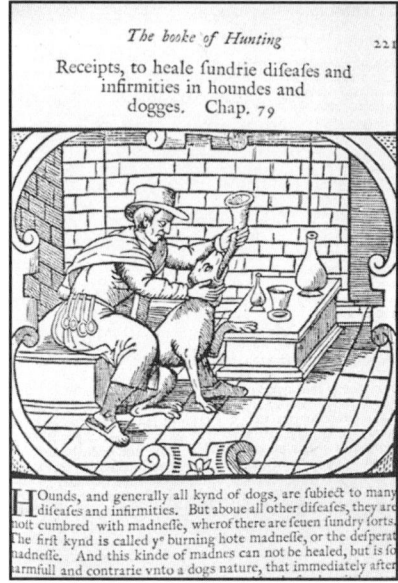

Turberville: Turbervile's booke of hunting,
1576, reprinted 1908 (1452)

1452. (**TURBERVILLE, George**) (1540-1610?). Turbervile's booke of hunting. **1908.** Oxford: Clarendon Press. Facsimile of 1576 ed, 250 pp. §

Reprint of a classic; includes dog diseases.

1453. **TUSON, Richard Vine** (1832-1888). A pharmacopoeia: including the outlines of materia medica and therapeutics for the use of practitioners and students of veterinary medicine. **1883.** Phila: P. Blakiston. 3rd ed, 358 pp.

From English work used at Royal Vet College.

1454. **TUSSER, Thomas** (1524?-1580). Five hundred points of good husbandry...together with a book of huswifery. **1810.** London: Lackington, Allen. 338 pp. §

A 16thC book (1st ed 1557) of poems including management of horses and diseases of cattle.

1455. **TUTTLE, S.A.** Veterinary experience: an invaluable treatise on the horse...diseases...remedies... **1897.** Boston: The author. 92 pp.

A promotion of the author's remedies.

1456. **UDALL, D(enny) H(ammond)** (1874-). The practice of veterinary medicine. **1933.** Ithaca, NY: The author. 267 pp. §

First edition of a standard work.

1457.__(same) **1943.** 743 pp. §

Sections on sulfonamides and allergy added.

1458.__(same) **1947.** 751 pp.

Includes use of penicillin and newer sulfa drugs.

1459.__Veterinarian's handbook of materia medica and therapeutics. **1912**. Ithaca, NY: Carpenter & Co. 177 pp. §
  Based on the author's practice experience.
1460. **UNDERHILL, Benjamin Mott.** Parasites and parasitosis of the domestic animals: the zoology and control of the animal parasites...and treatment of parasitic diseases. **1929**. New York: Macmillan. 379 pp. §
  A basic textbook with many illustrations.

United States Army Veterinary Service

1461.__Animal transport. War Department basic field manual. **1939**. Washington: GPO. 223 pp.
  The military system of horsemanship.
1462.__The army horse in accident and disease. A manual...for farriers and horseshoers...cavalry school, Fort Riley, KS. **1909**. Washington: GPO. 112 pp.
  On stable management and disease treatment.
1463.__Manual for stable sergeants...cavalry school, Fort Riley, KS. **1917**. Washington: GPO. 219 pp. §
  Emphasizes care of the foot; many illustrations.
1464.__Notes on equitation and horse training...School of Application for Cavalry at Saumur, France. **1910**. Washington: GPO. 98 pp. §
  On equitation for army officers.
1465.__Remount technical manual...War Department. **1941**. Washington: GPO. 99 pp.
  Regulations affecting army remount depots.
1466.__Veterinary bulletin. United States Army Veterinary Corps. Vol ll-35. **1923-41**. Carlisle Barracks, PA: Medical Field Service School.
1467.__The veterinary service. Army medical bulletin, No. 19. **1926**. Carlisle Barracks, PA: Medical Field Service School. 219 pp. §
  Organization and function of Army Vet Service.
1468.__Veterinary service regulations. **1921-34**. Carlisle Barracks, PA: Medical Field Service School. §
  Animal care, meat inspection, and other topics.

United States Department of Agriculture

1469.__Contagious diseases of domesticated animals...USDA special report No. 22. **1880**. Washington: GPO. 268 pp.
  Reports on swine plague, pleuropneumonia, rinderpest (cattle plague), Texas fever.
1470.__(same) Special report No. 36. **1881**. 391 pp. §
  Swine plague, fowl cholera, Texas fever, etc.

1471.___History of hog cholera research in the U.S. Department of Agriculture, 1884-1960. **1962.** Washington: GPO. 124 pp. §
   Chronology with emphasis on serum-vaccine use.
1472.___(same) **1962.** Supplement. 127 pp. §
1473.___Index-catalog of medical and veterinary zoology, compiled by A. Hassall, et al. **1932-52.** Washington: GPO. Parts 1-18 in 5 vol, 5711 pp.
   A monumental bibliography.
1474.___Investigations of diseases of swine, and infectious and contagious diseases incident to other classes of domesticated animals. **1879.** Washington: GPO. 292 pp. §
   Primarily swine plague; bovine pleuropneumonia.
1475.___Report of the Commissioner of Agriculture [extracts from]. Washington: GPO. 1865 (publ **1866**). pp 396-570. §
   Articles on cattle plague, dairying, feeding. Bound with:
1476.___(same) 1872 (publ **1874**). pp 203-348. §
   Equine influenza, milk sanitation, fish culture. Bound with:
1477.___(same) 1877 (publ **1878**). pp 333-528. §
   Articles on cattle breeding, hog cholera. Bound with:
1478.___(same) 1878 (publ **1879**). pp 321-476. §
   Articles on swine plague, glanders. Bound with:
1479.___(same) 1879 (publ **1880**). pp 365-484. §
   Swine plague, cattle plague, pleuropneumonia.
1480.___Report of the Commissioner of Agriculture [extracts from]. Washington: GPO. 1880 (publ **1881**). pp 387-608. §
   Swine plague, foot-and-mouth disease, Texas fever, pleuropneumonia, fowl cholera. Bound with:
1481.___(same) 1881-82 (publ **1882**). pp 257-377. §
   Swine plague, fowl cholera, Texas fever. Bound with:
1482.___(same) 1883 (publ **1883**). pp 17-81. §
   Articles on Texas fever, fowl cholera. Bound with:
1483.___(same) 1884 (publ **1884**). pp 181-284. §
   Ergotism, pleuropneumonia, Texas fever, gapeworm.
1484.___Report of the Commissioner of Agriculture. **1885.** Washington: GPO. 640 pp. §
   BAI reports on pleuropneumonia, swine plague, Texas fever and verminous bronchitis.
1485.___Report on the diseases of cattle in the United States, made to the Commissioner of Agriculture... **1869.** Washington: GPO. 190 pp. §
   Reports on pleuropneumonia, Texas fever.
1486.___Report...on the diseases of cattle in the United States. **1871.** Washington: GPO. 205 pp. §
   Pleuropneumonia, Texas fever, fungus diseases.
1487.___Special report of diseases of swine and other domestic animals. **1879.** Washington: GPO. 278 pp. §
   Swine plague, rinderpest, glanders, etc.

1488.__Yearbooks for 1899 & 1908 [extracts bound together]. **1900; 1908.** Washington: GPO. §
   Articles on bovine tuberculosis.

USDA Bureau of Animal Industry

1489.__Hog cholera: its history, nature, and treatment, as determined by the inquiries and investigations of the Bureau of Animal Industry. **1889.** Washington: GPO. 197 pp.
   Includes early attempts at vaccination.
1490.__[Extract from report of the Commissioner of Agriculture] Report of the Chief of the Bureau of Animal Industry. 1885 (publ **1886**). Washington: GPO. pp 431-568. §
   Swine plague, Texas fever, pleuropneumonia. Bound with:
1491.__(same) 1886 (publ **1887**). pp 593-686. §
   Hog cholera, swine plague, pleuropneumonia. Bound with:
1492.__(same) 1887 (publ **1888**). pp 457-522. §
   Hog cholera, swine plague, pleuropneumonia. Bound with:
1493.__(same) 1888 (publ **1889**). pp 145-219. §
   Glanders, hog cholera, swine plague. Bound with:
1494.__(same) 1889 (publ **1890**). pp 49-110. §
   Tuberculosis, pleuropneumonia, hog cholera. Bound with:
1495.__(same) 1890 (publ **1891**). pp 75-132. §
   Cattle trade, infectious diseases, Texas fever. Bound with:
1496.__(same) 1891 (publ **1892**). pp 83-142. §
   Cattle trade, swine plague, pleuropneumonia. Bound with:
1497.__(same) 1892 (publ **1893**). pp 85-122. §
   Texas fever, pleuropneumonia.
1498.__Annual report of the Bureau of Animal Industry for the year... 1889-90 (publ **1891**). Washington: GPO. 503 pp. §
1499.__(same) 1891-92 (publ **1893**). 428 pp.§
1500.__(same) 1895-96 (publ **1897**). 362 pp.§
1501.__(same) 1897 (publ **1898**). 727 pp.
   Anthrax, sheep scab, cerebrospinal meningitis.
1502.__(same) 1898 (publ **1899**). 647 pp.
   Glanders, Texas fever, tuberculosis, hog cholera.
1503.__(same) 1899 (publ **1900**). 790 pp.
   Texas fever, dairying, maladie du coit.
1504.__(same) 1900 (publ **1901**). 642 pp.§
1505.__(same) 1901 (publ **1902**). 706 pp.
   Parasites, surra, goats, tuberculosis.
1506.__(same) 1902 (publ **1903**). 651 pp.
   Tuberculosis, foot-and-mouth disease, scab.
1507.__(same) 1903 (publ **1904**). 618 pp.
   Tuberculosis, hog cholera. J. McFadyean copy.

1508.__(same) 1904 (publ **1905**). 632 pp.
 Cornstalk disease, tuberculosis, parasitism.
1509.__(same) 1905 (publ **1907**). 364 pp.§
1510.__(same) 1906 (publ **1908**). 478 pp. §
1511.__(same) 1908 (publ **1910**). 502 pp.
 Meat inspection, foot-and-mouth disease.
1512.__(same) 1909 (publ **1911**). 407 pp.
 Surra, rabies, anthrax, cattle ticks.
1513.__(same) 1910 (publ **1912**). 573 pp.
 Texas fever, glanders, parasites, tuberculosis.
1514.__(same) 1911 (publ **1913**). 356 pp.
 Brucellosis, abortion, meat inspection.
1515.__Special report on diseases of cattle and on cattle feeding. **1892**. Washington: GPO. 496 pp.
 Written for cattle owners and practitioners, with chapters by noted veterinarians.
1516.__(same) **1896**. 496 pp. §
 Title changed on 1904 and later editions.
1517.__Special report on diseases of cattle. **1904**. Washington: GPO. 533 pp. §
 Extensively revised (and later re-revised).
1518.__(same) **1906**. [?]
1519.__(same) **1909**. 551 pp. §
1520.__(same) **1916**. 568 pp. §
1521.__(same) **1923**. 563 pp. §
1522.__(same) **1942**. 507 pp. §
1523.__Special report on diseases of the horse. **1890**. Washington: GPO. 556 pp. §
 Written and revised as for Diseases of cattle.
1524.__(same) **1896**. 576 pp. §
1525.__(same) **1903**. 600 pp.
1526.__(same) **1907**. 608 pp. §
1527.__(same) **1911**. 614 pp. §
1528.__(same) **1916**. 629 pp. §
1529.__(same) **1923**. 629 pp. §
1530.__(same) **1942**. 584 pp. §
1531.__Special report on the history and present condition of the sheep industry of the United States. **1892**. Washington: GPO. 1000 pp. §
 On sheep breeds and husbandry.

1532. **URQUHART, David** (1805-1877). Manual of the Turkish bath: heat a mode of cure and a source of strength for men and animals. **1865**. London: John Churchill. 419 pp. §
 With a minor section on horses and cattle.
1533. **VAN ES, L.; HARRIS, E.D.; SCHALK, A.F.** Swamp fever in horses. North Dakota AES Bulletin 94. **1911**. Fargo: ND AES. 96 pp.

1534. **VAN MATER, George G.** (1863-). A text book of veterinary ophthalmology. **1897.** New York: W.R. Jenkins. 157 pp. §
  A text antedating the teaching of this subject.

1535. **VAN OLINDA, H.** A new system of horse training, including a treatise on shoeing. **1865.** Albany, NY: Van Benthuysen. 31 pp.
  A pamphlet promising more than it delivers.

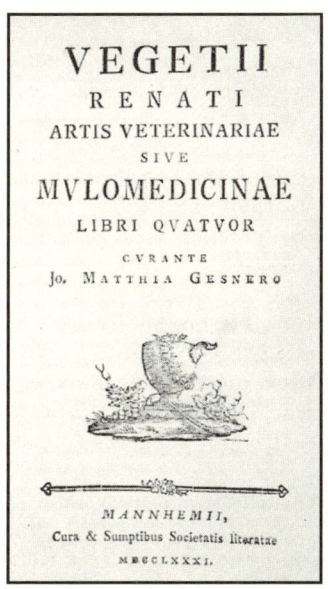
Vegetius: 1781 (793) (1536)

1536. **VEGETIUS RENATUS, Publius** (fl 450-500 AD). Of the distempers of horses, and of the art of curing them. **1748.** London: A. Millar. 421 pp. §
  A translation of: "Books of the veterinary art" (5thC) written by an enlightened layman.

1537. **VESEY-FITZGERALD, Brian Seymour** (1900-). The book of the horse. **1947.** London: Nicholson & Watson. 879 pp. §
  History, breeds, breeding, and the horse in art and literature; copiously illustrated.

1538. __The domestic dog: an introduction to its history. **1957.** London: Routledge & K. Paul. 226 pp. §
  Domestication and the dog in art, literature, etc.

Veterinary Associations

1539. __The Alabama VMA: 75 years of organized service. **1982.** [s.l.]: Alabama VMA. 50 pp.
  Includes history of schools (Auburn, Tuskegee).

1540.__American Animal Hospital Association. 50 years of educational excellence and practice improvement. **1983.** Mishawaka, IN: AAHA. 64 pp. §

The first 50 years; copiously illustrated.

1541.__AAHA. Proceedings of the third annual meeting. **1936.** Evanston, IL: AAHA. 64 pp. §

Papers on rabies, anesthesia, hospitals, etc.

1542.__AAHA. Proceedings of the fourth annual meeting (1937). **1938.** Evanston, IL: AAHA. 110 pp. §

Radiology, eye, thyroid, surgery, neurology, etc.

1543.__AAHA. Proceedings of the fifth annual meeting. **1938.** Evanston, IL: AAHA. 77 pp. §

Anesthesia, parasites, kidney, gastritis, etc.

1544.__USVMA (predecessor of AVMA). Proceedings of the United States Veterinary Medical Association, 1893 (publ **1894**). Phila: USVMA. 381 pp.

Papers on vet history, education, Texas fever, hog cholera, fistula, pleuropneumonia, etc.

1545.__(same) **1896.** Phila: USVMA. 240 pp.

Horseshoeing, dentistry, TB, hog cholera, etc. S.B. Nelson signature.

1546.__(same) **1897.** Kansas City: USVMA. 272 pp.

Osteoporosis, education, pneumonia, rabies, etc.

1547.__(same) **1898.** Ithaca, NY: USVMA. 212 pp. §

Meat inspection, disinfection, indigestion, roaring, hog cholera, Texas fever, etc.

1548.__Proceedings of the American Veterinary Medical Association. **1899.** Ithaca, NY: AVMA. 304 pp.§

Anesthesia, azoturia, milk hygiene, milk fever, tetanus, rabies, tuberculosis, etc.

1549.__(same) **1900.** St Paul: Pioneer Press. 296 pp. §

Scabies, rabies, azoturia, tuberculosis, etc.

1550.__(same) **1901.** St Paul: Webb Publ. 408 pp. §

Anthrax, canine distemper, disinfection, TB, etc.

1551.__(same) **1902.** St Paul: Pioneer Press. 346 pp. §

Poisoning, milk fever, shipping fever, Tx fever.

1552.__(same) **1903.** 346 pp. §

Tumors, encephalitis, parasites, glanders, TB.

1553.__(same) **1904.** Hartford, CN: Hartford Press. 410 pp. §

Glanders, education, surgery, blood, mange, TB.

1554.__(same) **1905.** 506 pp. §

Glanders, lameness, blood, neurotomy, surgery.

1555.__(same) **1906.** Phila: AVMA. 427 pp. §

Roaring, rabies, glanders, mange, etc.

1556.__(same) **1907.** Phila: J.B. Lippincott. 555 pp. §

Tumors, milk hygiene, roaring, education, TB.

1557.__(same) **1908.** 466 pp. §

Public health, Texas fever, glanders, history, shipping fever, milk hygiene, etc.

1558.__(same) 1909 (publ **1910**). 413 pp. §

Infectious anemia, Texas fever, milk hygiene, TB.

1559.__(same) 1910 (publ **1911**). Lansing, MI: R. Smith. 522 pp. §
Dourine, anesthesia, surgery, milk hygiene, TB.
1560.__(same) **1911**. 725 pp. §
Roaring, spaying, hog cholera, abortion, anthrax glanders, pneumonia, hematuria, etc.
1561.__(same) 1912 (publ **1913**). 719 pp. §
Lameness, reproduction, ophthalmia, hog cholera, glanders, education, etc; J.V. Lacroix signature.
1562.__(same) 1913 (publ **1914**). Phila: W.J. Dornan. 1084 pp. §
Mastitis, meningitis, artificial insemination, spaying, colic, roaring, lameness, firing, etc.
1563.__British Veterinary Association issue. Veterinary Record. **1982**. Vol 110, No. 26. §
Several papers related to BVA centennial.
1564.__Indiana VMA. Proceedings of annual meeting. **1913**. Lafayette, IN: IVMA. 32 pp. §
1565.__(same) **1935-36**. Indianapolis: IVMA. 194 pp. §
Papers on anesthesia, blood transfusion, hog cholera, public health, breeding, etc.
1566.__Eastern Iowa Veterinary Association. 25th anniversary souvenir book, 1913-1938. **1939**. NP: The assn. 155 pp. §
With many portraits and biographies.
1567.__New York City Veterinary Medical Association. Constitution and bylaws. **1891**. 10 pp.
1568.__New York State Veterinary Medical Society. Constitution and bylaws. **1937**. 11 pp.

Veterinary Colleges

1569.__(Alfort) Deuxieme centenaire de l'ecole nationale veterinaire d'Alfort. **1967**. Paris: Receuil de Med Vet. Vol 143, No. 11, pp 1031-1212. §
Bicentennial of the Alfort school, with a homage to Gaston Ramon.
1570.__(Cornell) New York State Veterinary College. Addresses and papers...for the years 1896-1898. **1898**. Ithaca, NY: Cornell Univ. 606 pp. §
1571.__Don't forget the horse doctor [James Law]. The first forty years of one of the first veterinary colleges in America. **1980**. Ithaca, NY: Office of Univ Publ. 28 pp. §
An illustrated history of the veterinary college.
1572.__(Cornell) Society of comparative medicine of the New York State Veterinary College. Program, second annual banquet. **1905**. Ithaca, NY: [s.n.] 25 pp. §
In honor of James Law.
1573.__Kansas City Veterinary College. Official history and directory. **1956**. [s.l. s.n.] 29 pp. §
Listings of faculty and students 1892-1918.

1574.__(same) Pictorial review. **1915.** Kansas City: KCVC. 48 pp. §
   Numerous photos of facilities and equipment.
1575.__(London) An account of the veterinary college from its institution in 1791. **1793.** London: James Phillips. 77 pp. §
   Includes college rules and list of subscribers.
1576.__(Michigan State University) MSC [MSU] Veterinarian. **1953.** Vol 13, No. 3. Dedication issue. §
   Includes history of veterinary medicine at MSU.
1577.__Royal (Dick) Veterinary College. Prospectus. **1889-90.** Edinburgh: The college. 62 pp. §
   Includes entrance examinations.
1578.__(same) **1896-97.** 110 pp. §
1579.__(same) **1897-98.** 115 pp. §
   With 39-p supplement (separate).
1580.__(University of Pennsylvania) History of the School of Veterinary Medicine of the University of Pennsylvania, 1884-1934...fiftieth anniversary... **1935.** Phila: Vet Alumni Soc. 226 pp. §
   Includes lists of faculty and graduates.
1581.__(same) The veterinary profession: its relation to the health and wealth of the nation, and what it offers as a career... **1897.** Phila: [s.n.] 83 pp. §
   Short articles by faculty and alumni.
1582.__(Universita di Torino) Bicentenario della facolta di medicina veterinaria, 1769-1969. **1969.** Torino: [s.n.] 364 pp.
   Bicentennial volume of the school at Turin.
1583.__United States College of Veterinary Surgeons. Catalog. **1917.** Washington: The college. 42 pp. §
   Curriculum and description of courses.

Veterinary History

1584.__American Veterinary History Society Newsletter. **1976-82.** Santa Barbara, CA; Fort Dodge, IA: The society. 7 issues. Continued as:
1585.__Veterinary Heritage ; Bulletin of the American Veterinary History Society. **1982-.** Pullman, WA; Ames. IA: The society. Vol 6-.
1586.__Cornell Veterinarian, 75th anniversary issue. **1985.** Ithaca, NY. Vol 75, No. 1. §
   20 papers on past, present and future.
1587.__Historia Medicina Veterinariae. **1976-.** Copenhagen: Amici HMV. Vol 1-.
   Vol 1-10 bound; vol 11 unbound.
1588.__Journal of the American Veterinary Medical Association. Diamond jubilee number. **1938.** Chicago: AVMA. Vol 92, No. 6. §
   Several articles on early vet med in America.

1589.__(same) US bicentennial issue. **1976.** Schaumburg, IL: AVMA. Vol 169, No. 1. §
   15 papers on history of vet med in America.
1590.__MD: medical newsmagazine. Veterinary medicine issue. **1975.** New York: MD Publ. October. §
   Feature article and others on veterinary history.
1591.__Medical Heritage. Veterinary medicine issue. **1986.** Phila: W.B. Saunders. July/Aug. §
   Several articles on veterinary history.
1592.__MSU Veterinarian. Veterinary history issue. **1960.** East Lansing, MI: [s.n.]. Fall. §
   18 articles on veterinary history.
1593.__Veterinary History: Bulletin of the Veterinary History Society. **1973-.** London: The society.
   Old series No. 1-12 (1979-83); n.s. Vol 1-.
1594.__Veterinary Medicine. 50th anniversary issue. **1955.** Kansas City: Vet Med Publ Co. Vol 50. No. 11. §
   Several papers on veterinary history.

Veterinary Periodicals

1595.__American Journal of Veterinary Medicine. **1912-17.** Chicago: Vet Med Publ Co. Vol 7, 9-12. §
   Supersedes Missouri Valley Vet Bulletin; superseded by Veterinary Medicine.
1596.__American Veterinary Journal. **1851/52** (old series) Vol 1; **1855/56; 1858/59.** (n.s.) Vol 1-4. Boston: G.H. Dadd.
   First true veterinary periodical in America.
1597.__(same) **1855.** n.s. Vol 1, No. 1. (facsimile) §
   First article on anesthesia in US vet jnl.
1598.__American Veterinary Review. **1877-1915.** New York: A. Liautard (to 1898). Vol 1-47.
   Acquired by AVMA in 1915 and became JAVMA.
1599.__Edinburgh Veterinary Review and Annals of Comparative Pathology. **1858-64.** Edinburgh: Sutherland & Knox. Vol 1-6.
1600.__The Journal of Comparative Medicine and Veterinary Archives. **1880-93.** New York: W.L. Hyde. Vol 1-24.
1601.__Missouri Valley Veterinary Bulletin. **1909-10.** Vol 4, No 1-12. §
1602.__The Veterinarian: a monthly journal of veterinary science. **1828-1902.** London: Longman, Rees. Vol 1-75.
   William Percivall and William Youatt, first eds.
1603.__Veterinary Journal and Annals of Comparative Pathology. **1875-1899.** London: Bailliere, Tindall. Vol 1-49. (lacks several volumes).

1604.__The Veterinary Record, and Transactions of the Veterinary Medical Association. **1845-50**. London: Longman, Brown. Vol 1-6.
Superseded by Veterinary Record.
1605.__Veterinary Standard. **1913-16**. Grand Rapids, MI: Grand Rapids Veterinary College. Vol 3-6. §
Lacks some numbers in each volume.

Vial de St Bel—see Sainbel, Vial de

1606. **VINES, Richard.** A practical treatise on glanders and farcy in the horse. **1830**. London: Longman, Rees. 208 pp.
Erroneous views on cause and treatment.
1607. **(VIRGIL).** The complete works of Virgil. Trans by C. Day Lewis. **1947**. New York: Oxford Univ Press. 83 pp. §
Perceptive writings (1stC BC) on animal disease, including mange and anthrax; horse breeding.
1608. **VOGEL, Eduard.** Spezielle Arzneimittellehre fur Tierarzte. **1886**. Stuttgart: Paul Neff. 3rd ed, 688 pp.
Mainly a materia medica and pharmacopoeia.
1609. **VOGEL, Virgil J.** American Indian medicine. **1970**. Norman: Univ Oklahoma Press. 584 pp. §
Includes references to veterinary medicine.
1610. **WADDELL, William H.** The black man in veterinary medicine. **1969**. Fargo. ND: [s.n.] 56 pp.
Tribulations and achievements of blacks.
1611.__(same) **1982**. [s.l. s.n.] 176 pp.
1612.__People are the funniest animals. **1978**. Phila: Dorrance. 329 pp.
Anecdotal biography of early black AVMA member.
1613.__Universal veterinarianism. **1973**. [s.l. s.n.] 114 pp.
Bits about the colleges and blacks in vet med.
1614. **WALKER, Robin E.** Ars veterinaria: l'art veterinaire de l'antiquite a la fin du XIXeme siecle: essai historique. **1972**. Levallois-Perret, Galena. 85 pp. §
A brief history, beautifully illustrated.
1615. **WALSH, John Henry** (1810-1888). The dog in health and disease: comprising the various modes of breaking and using him for hunting, coursing...by Stonehenge [pseud.]. **1887**. London: Longmans, Green. 4th ed, 412 pp. §
On breeds, management and disease treatment.
1616.__The dogs of Great Britain, America, and other countries. Their breeding, training, and management in health and disease... **1919**. New York: O. Judd. 369 pp. §
A standard work, with good section on diseases.
1617.__The horse in the stable and the field: his management and disease...with additions by Robert McClure... **1871**. Phila: Porter & Coates. 540 pp. §
From London ed; extensive section on disease.

1618.__(same) **1882**. 505 pp. §
1619.__The horse: its varieties and management in health and disease. **1880**? London: F. Warne. 259 pp. §
   Disease section mainly on inflammation.
1620. **WALTHER, Johan.** Kurze Beschreibung der Pferde-und Vieh-zucht... **1658**. [s.l.]: C. von Saher. 127 pp.
   Diseases of horses, cattle and sheep, with 23 pp manuscript receipt book at front of book.
1621. **WARD, Archibald Robinson** (1875-). Diseases of domesticated birds. **1922**. New York: Macmillan. 459 pp. §
   Includes canaries and the ostrich.
1622. **WARD, William.** A new treatise on the method of breeding, breaking, and training horses. **1776**. Edinburgh: Dickson, Elliot. 200 pp. §
   Ingenious training method; worthless on disease.
1623. **WARE, Jean.** The several lives of a Victorian vet. **1980**. New York: St Martins's Press. 213 pp.
   Biography of Griffith Evans, dubbed "father" of veterinary science in Great Britain.
1624.**WARLOMONT, Evariste** (1820-1899). A manual of animal vaccination preceded by consideration of vaccination in general. Trans by A.J. Harries. **1886**. Phila: J. Wyeth. 152 pp.
   Propagation of vaccines in animals, for humans.
1625. **WATERMAN, George Arthur.** The practical stock doctor: compiled from the most successful veterinarians in the world... **1908**. Detroit: F.B. Dickerson. 808 pp. §
   Text for farmers; remedies of dubious value.
1626.__The practical stock doctor: a reliable, common-sense ready-reference book. **1912**. Detroit: F.B. Dickerson. 840 pp. §
   Like 1908 ed, with 32 pp of illustrations.
1627.__The practical stock doctor: the farmer's short courses in live stock... **1920**. Detroit; Windsor, Ontario: F.B. Dickerson. 960 pp. §
   Like 1912 ed, with index of symptoms added; correspondence course certificate included.
1628.__The practical stock doctor: course II. Cattle, sheep, hogs and poultry. **1920**. Detroit: F.B. Dickerson. 286 pp. §
1629.__(same) **1921**. Lincoln, NE: F.B. Dickerson. 286 pp. §
1630. **WATSON, Thomas, Sir** (1792-1882). Lectures on the principles and practice of physic. Delivered at King's College, London. **1845**. Phila: Lea & Blanchard. 2nd American ed. 1060 pp. §
   Includes use of curare for tetanus at London Vet College; section on rabies in man and dog.
1631. **WEBSTER, Leslie Tillotson** (1894-). Rabies. **1942**. New York: Macmillan. 168 pp. §
   A definitive work on the subject.

1632. **WEDL, Carl** (1815-1891). Rudiments of pathological histology. Trans by George Busk. **1855**. London: Sydenham Society. 637 pp. §
Includes diseases of veterinary interest.

1633. **WEISS, C.F.H.** Specielle Physiologie der Haussaugethiere fur Thierarzte... **1869**. Stuttgart: J.D. Metzler. 547 pp.
Introductory physiology of domestic animals.

1634. **WELLS, Ellen B.** Horsemanship: a bibliography of printed materials from the sixteenth century through 1974. **1985**. New York: Garland Publ. 282 pp.
With 8500 items, many of veterinary interest.

1635. **WHARTON, Charles.** Hand-book on the treatment of the horse in the stable and on the road... **1873**. Phila: J.B. Lippincott. 137 pp. §
With details of diagnosis of foot lameness.

1636. **WHITE, David Stuart** (1869-1944). A textbook of the principles and practice of veterinary medicine. **1917**. Phila; New York: Lea & Febiger. 484 pp.
By the dean of vet med at Ohio State Univ.

1637. **WHITE, George Ransom.** Animal castration. **1947**. Nashville, TN: The author. 3rd ed, 287 pp. §
A long-standard work (1st ed 1917); illustrated.

1638.__Restraint of domestic animals: a book for the use of students and practitioners. **1909**. Nashville, TN: The author. 302 pp. §
A comprehensive work; copiously illustrated.

1639.__(same) **1912**. 2nd ed, 302 pp. §

James White (-1825)

1640.__A compendious dictionary of the veterinary art: containing a concise explanation of the various terms used in veterinary medicine and surgery... **1817**. London: Longman, Hurst. 344 pp. §
Differs from other works with similar titles, which make White the bane of bibliographers.

1641.__A compendium of cattle medicine...the disorders of cattle and other domestic animals, except the horse... **1823**. Phila: Carey & Lea. 233 pp.
A reissue of his "Treatise," vol 4 (qv).

1642.__(same) **1842**. London: Longman, Brown. 6th ed, with additions by W.C. Spooner. 322 pp.

1643.__A compendium of the veterinary art...the diseases to which the horse is liable, their symptoms and treatment... **1802**. Canterbury: J. Badcock. 232 pp.

1644.__(same)...the disorders and accidents to which the horse is liable... **1822**. London: Longman, Hurst. 13th ed, 348 pp.
Uneven; good in some areas, weak in others.

1645.__(same) **1829**. London: Longman, Rees. 15th ed, 340 pp. §

1646.__(same)...construction and management of the stable...structure and economy of the horse. **1842**. London: Longman, Brown. 17th ed, 558 pp. §
With extensive pharmacopoeia by W.C Spooner.

1647.__(same) **1851**. 18th ed, 560 pp. §

1648.__A complete system of farriery and veterinary medicine: containing a compendium of the veterinary art... **1818**. Pittsburgh: Patterson & Lambdin. 1st American ed, from 10th London ed, 311 pp. §

An early work published in the "western" US.

1649.__(same) **1832**. Pittsburgh: H. Holdship. 2nd American ed, 216 pp. §

1650.__The improved art of farriery...structure and economy of the horse...management of the stable...symptoms, and treatment of all diseases... **1857**. London: H.G. Bohn. 619 pp.

A disorganized compilation, with no improvement.

1651.__A treatise on veterinary medicine. **1808-09**. London: Longman, Hurst. 9th ed, 2 vol in 1; 409; 266 pp.

Based on London Veterinary College teaching.

1652.__(same) London: Longman, Hurst. 4 vol. Vol 1 (essentially 9th ed Compendium) **1812**. 370 pp; Vol 2 (pharmacopoeia, as for item 1651, vol 2) **1811**. 266 pp; Vol 3 (mainly on diseases of horses) **1812**. 262 pp; Vol 4 (diseases of cattle, sheep, swine) **1815**. 204 pp.

"A worthless jumble." (Smith)

1653.__(same) **1823**. London: Longman, Hurst. Vol 2. 4th ed, 329 pp. §

As for 1811 ed, with materia dietetica added.

1654.__(same) **1823**. London: Longman, Hurst. Vol 3. 6th ed, 384 pp. §

1655.__(same) **1825**. Vol 3. 7th ed, 384 pp.

Same as 6th ed.

1656.__(same) **1830**. London: Longman, Rees. Vol 3. 8th ed, 384 pp. §

1657.__(same) **1831**. London: Longman, Rees. Vol 2. 6th ed, 360 pp. §

1658.(__) The farrier's guide. **1756**. London: J.B. [?]

Erroneously attributed to White, who qualified at London in 1797. (Smith)

1659. **WHITEHEAD, G. Kenneth.** The ancient white cattle of Britain and their descendants. **1953**. London: Faber & Faber. 174 pp. §

Description of herds, ancient and modern.

1660. **WIGMORE, William, H.** Practical caponizing and how to make poultry pay... **1886**. Phila: Franklin News.

A pamphlet including poultry management.

1661. **WILKINSON, Lise.** Animals and diseases: an introduction to the history of comparative medicine. **1992**. Cambridge: Cambridge Univ Press. 272 pp. §

Impact of cattle plague and veterinary schools on development of 18th-19thC medicine/vet med.

1662. **WILLEMS, Le Docteur.** Etat de la question de l'inoculation de la pleuropneumonie exsudative de l'espece bovine en 1861. **1861**. Hasselt: H.J. Ceysens. 23 pp.

1663. **WILLIAMS, C.H.C.** Williams' new system of handling and educating the horse: together with diseases and their treatment... **1880**. Claremont, NH: Claremont Mfg Co. 331 pp. §

A little information on a lot of subjects.

1664. **WILLIAMS, Mrs Leslie.** The cat: its care and management. **1908.** Phila: H. Altemus. 219 pp. §
Owner's handbook; includes diseases.

1665. **WILLIAMS, Walter Long** (1856-1945). The diseases of the genital organs of domestic animals. **1921.** Ithaca, NY: The author. 856 pp. §
A classic work by a noted theriogenologist.

1666.__(same) **1943.** 3rd ed, 641 pp. §

1667.__Surgical and obstetrical operations, for veterinary students and practitioners... **1903.** Ithaca, NY: The author. 210 pp. §
Handbook of technics for surgical exercises.

1668.__(same) **1912.** 3rd ed, 240 pp. §

1669.__Veterinary obstetrics, including the diseases of breeding animals and of the new-born. **1909.** Ithaca, NY: The author. 1127 pp. §
Later separated into 2 works (items 1665; 1670).

1670.__Veterinary obstetrics. **1943.** Ithaca, NY: The author. 478 pp. §
Presentation copy to J.V. Lacroix.

William Williams

1671.__The principles and practice of veterinary medicine. **1874.** Edinburgh: MacLachlan & Stewart. 704 pp.
An early work based on scientific principles.

1672.__(same) **1879.** New York: William Wood. 2nd ed, 768 pp.

1673.__(same) **1892.** New York: W.R. Jenkins. Rev ed, 590 pp. §
Numerous plates added, some in color.

1674.__(same) **1893.** Rev by author and his son, W. Owen Williams. 7th ed, 838 pp. §

1675.__(same) **1893.** New ed, 590 pp. §

1676.__(same) **1897.** Edinburgh: John Menzies. Rev by author and his son. 3rd ed, 863 pp.

1677.__The principles and practice of veterinary surgery. **1882.** New York: W.R. Jenkins. 4th ed, 740 pp. §
A standard text with emphasis on the horse.

1678.__(same) **1891.** New York: Sabiston & Murray. Special American ed, 756 pp.

1679. **WILSON, Yorick.** The gentleman's veterinary monitor and stable guide: a concise treatise on the various diseases of horses... **1809.** London: Bone & Hone. 123 pp.
"A worthless and ignorant product." (Smith)

1680. **WINDISCH-GRAETZ, Mathilde.** The Spanish riding school: its traditions and development... **1955?** New York: A.S. Barnes. 35 pp text, 80 plates. §
The history and training of the Lippizaner stud.

1681. **WINSLOW, Kenelm** (1863-). The prevention and treatment of diseases of the domestic animals... **1910.** New York: W.R. Jenkins. 303 pp.
Emphasizes etiology as basis of prevention.

1682.___Veterinary materia medica and therapeutics. **1902.** New York: W.R. Jenkins. 2nd ed, 755 pp.
   A standard text for many years.
1683.___(same) **1906.** 4th ed, 804 pp.
   J.E. McCoy signature.
1684.___(same) **1913.** 7th ed, 779 pp. §
1685.___(same) **1916.** 7th ed, 781 pp.
   E.A. Ehmer signature.
1686.___(same) **1919.** Chicago: Amer Vet Publ Co. 8th ed, 640 pp. §
   With chapter on biologics by A. Eichhorn.
1687. **WINTER, Georg Simon** (1634?-). Pferde-Arzt: welcher grundlich lehret, wie man...alle innerlichen und ausserlichen Krankheiten curiren... **1757.** Nurnberg: J.A. Endter. 838 pp. §
   Treatment of equine diseases, with many Rx.

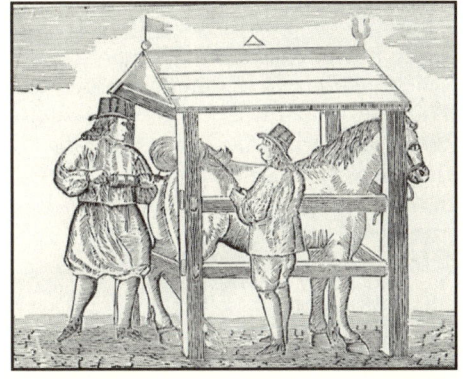

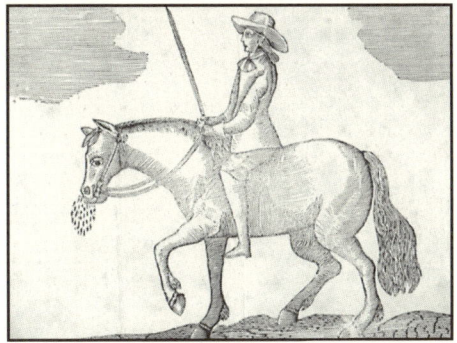

Winter: Pferde-Arzt, 1840 (1688)

1688.___(same) **1840.** Phila: E.Y. Schelly. 838 pp. §
   Reprint in smaller format, with folding plates.

1689. **WINTER, James W.** The horse, in health and disease...varieties, conformation...training, and shoeing...with a digest of veterinary practice. **1846.** London: Longman, Brown. 376 pp. §
  Good on management and shoeing; well-written.
1690. **WOOD, H.C.; REMINGTON, J.P.; SADTLER, S.P.** The dispensatory of the United States of America. **1899.** Phila: J.B. Lippincott. 2091 pp. §
  Index contains some 20,000 entries.
1691. **WOOD, John.** A new compendious treatise of farriery...the disorders incident to horses and their respective cures... **1757.** London: The author. 334 pp. §
  By a groom who knew nothing of the subject.
1692. **(WOOD, Mary S.)** (1805-1894). Canary birds. A manual of useful and practical information for bird keepers. **1866.** New York: W. Wood. 110 pp. §
  Includes a short section on diseases.
1693. **WOODVILLE, William** (1752-1805). Reports of a series of inoculations for the variola vaccina, or cow-pox... **1799.** London: J. Phillips. 156 pp.
  Early history of vaccination, with case reports.
1694. **WRANGEL, Carl Gustav.** Das Buch vom Pferde: ein Handbuch... **1890.** Stuttgart: Schickhardt & Ebner. 2 vol, 639; 596 pp.
  Horse management, with brief section on disease.
1695. **WYMAN, W(illy) E(dward) A(lexander).** The clinical diagnosis of lameness in the horse. **1898.** New York: W.R. Jenkins. 171 pp. §
  Based on the teachings of Heinrich Moller.
1696. **(XENOPHON).** The whole works of Xenophon. Trans by Ashley Cooper et al. **1851.** New York: R. Carter. 758 pp. §
  Includes work (4thC BC) on horsemanship.

William Youatt (1776-1847)

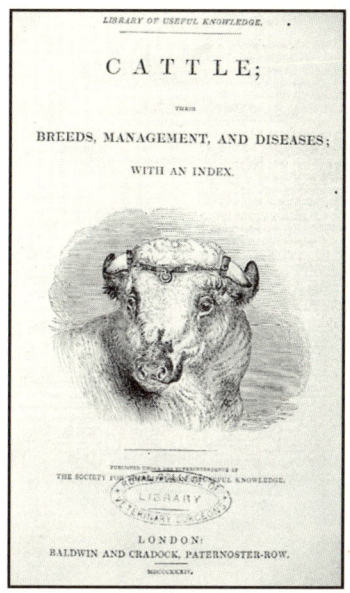

Youatt: 1834 (1697)

1697.___Cattle: their breeds, management, and diseases... **1834**. London: R. Baldwin. 600 pp. §
   A scholarly work by a noted veterinarian.
1698.___The dog. **1886**. London: Longmans, Green. 270 pp.
   A classic work on dog breeds and disease.
1699.___(same) **1890**. London; New York: Longmans, Green. 270 pp.
1700.___(same) **1848**. Edited with additions by E.J. Lewis. Phila: Lea & Blanchard. 403 pp. §
1701.___(same) **1879**. Phila: J.B. Lippincott. 403 pp. §
1702.___The horse: with a treatise on draught. **1848**. London: Charles Knight. New ed (1st ed 1831), 581 pp. §
   A classic work on breeds, anatomy and disease.
1703.___(same) **1872**. Boston; New York: Lee, Shephard. 4th ed, 589 pp. §
1704.___(same) **1880?** With an appendix, intended to advance the work to the present state of veterinary science, by W.C. Spooner. London: R. Baldwin. 529 pp.
1705.___(same) **1898**. Edited by Walker Watson. London: Longmans, Green. 589 pp.
1706.___The horse: with a general history of the horse: a dissertation on the American trotting horse ...and an essay on the ass and mule, by J.S. Skinner. **1843**. New York: Leavitt & Allen. 448 pp. §
   Disease sections largely from English edition.

1707.__(same) **1843**. Phila: Lea & Blanchard. 448 pp. §

1708.__The pig. **1860**. Rev by Samuel Sidney. Comprising modern pigs, breeding, feeding...medical information...London; New York: Routledge, Warne. 260 pp. §

A major revision of a standard British work.

1709.__Sheep: their breeds, management, and diseases... **1837**. London: R. Baldwin. 368 + 36 pp.

With The mountain shepherd's manual added.

1710.__(same) **1848**. New York: O. Judd. 159 pp. §

Section on sheep management in the US added.

1711.__(same) **1848**. New York: A.O. Moore. 159 pp.

Bound with: Randall: Sheep husbandry (qv).

1712.__(same) **1855**. New York: C.M. Saxton. 160 pp.

1713.__; **MARTIN, W.C.L.** Cattle : being a treatise on their breeds, management, and diseases... **1851**. New York: C.M. Saxton. 469 pp.

An abridgement of the British edition.

1714.__(same) **1859**. New York: A.O. Moore. 469 pp. §

1715.__(same) **1881**. New York: O. Judd. 470 pp.

1716.(__) A history of the horse, in all its varieties and uses : together with...the cure of all diseases to which he is liable. Also a concise treatise on draught... **1834**. Washington: D. Green. 360 pp. §

An anonymous abridged plagiary; much verbatim.

1717.(__) Youatt on the structure and the diseases of the horse...being the most important parts of the English edition... **1860**. New York: O. Judd. 483 pp. §

1718.(__) (same) **1850**. Auburn, NY: Derby & Miller 483 pp. §

1719.(__) (same) **1851**. New York: Derby & Miller. 483 pp.

1720.(__) (same) **1854**. Auburn, NY: Miller, Orton. 483 pp. §

1721.(__) (same) **1857**. New York: Miller, Orton. 483 pp.

1722.(__) (same) **1860**. New York: C.M. Saxton. 483 pp. §

1723.(__) Youatt's history, treatment, and diseases of the horse: embracing...general management under all peculiar circumstances... **1860**. Phila: J.B. Lippincott. 470 pp. §

1724.(__) (same) **1875**. 470 pp. §

1725. **YOUNG, Martin.** M. Young's new guide to horse owners : and complete horse doctor. **1880?**. New York: The author. 98 pp. §

1726.__(same) **1940?** 104 pp. §

1727. **YOUNG, Wesley A.** (1898-); **MIKLOWITZ, Gloria D.** The zoo was my world. **1969**. New York: Dutton. 128 pp.

Memoirs of a Los Angeles zoo veterinarian, with W.A. Young signature.

1728. **ZUEND, Johann Joseph.** Handbuch der Pferde- und Vieharzney-Kunde...innerliche Krankheiten... **1832**. Phila: The author. 376 pp. §

1729.__(same) **1834**. 376 pp. §

Appendix

A001. **ADVERTISING AND PROMOTION.** Flyers, booklets, cards, etc, 19th-early 20thC. (7 items, including Barker's "Komic" Picture Souvenir, Pt 1. The Barker, Moore & Mein Medicine Co, Phila, ca 1900. Promoting Barker's veterinary medicines with comic cartoons.) §

A002. **AMBULANCES, Animal.** Illustrations, reprints. (5 items) §
See also: Military, World War I.

A003. **AMERICAN ANIMAL HOSPITAL ASSOCIATION.** Records, 1933-82. §

___ (a). Executive Board minutes, 1933-55. Typescript (photocopy), ca 100 pp.

___ (b). Annual meeting programs, 1934-59. Photocopies.

___ (c). History, as related by Mark Morris, Nov. 1974. Typescript (photocopy), 16 pp.

___ (d). Mark Morris. Transcript of interview with Morris, first president of AAHA, by David Drennan, July 1982. Typescript with autograph corrections. 55 pp.

A004. **ASPCA.** Newburgh, NY Branch. Records, 1976-82. §

___ (a). Scrapbook, 1976-82. Minutes of meetings, treasurer's reports, correspondence, etc.

___ (b). Letters (5): 2 autograph letters signed from Henry Bergh, president ASPCA, to Peter Eager, first president Newburgh branch, 1876, 1880; 1 autograph letter signed to Eager from Thomas Hartfield of ASPCA 1879; 2 autograph letters signed from L.B. Wood, veterinary surgeon, of Newburgh, 1876, 1877.

A005. **AMERICAN VETERINARY PROFESSION.** (9 items) §

A006. **ANIMAL WELFARE.** (3 Items) Mainly vivisection. §

A007. **ASSOCIATION FOR WOMEN VETERINARIANS.** Records, 1947-. The records of the Association (formerly Women's Veterinary Medical Assn), consisting of correspondence, financial records, general (minutes, registers), printed materials (bulletins, etc), and scrapbooks. The collection is open-ended, ie, records continue to be added on a regular basis. See also: Women Veterinarians.

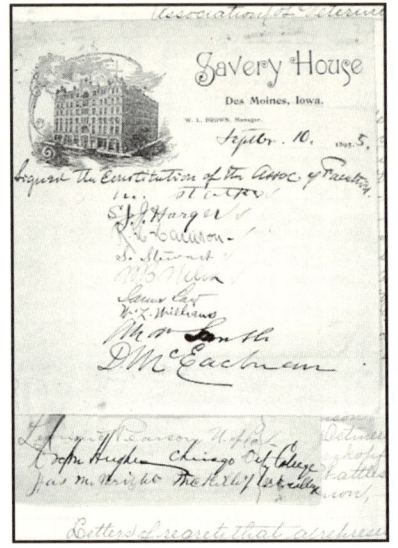 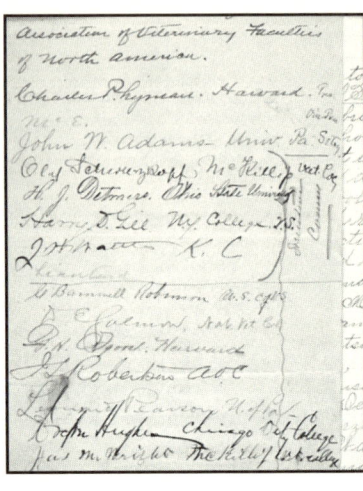

Association of veterinary faculties of North America: Minute book. Signatures of charter members, 1895 (A008)

A008. **ASSOCIATION OF VETERINARY FACULTIES (and Examining Boards) OF NORTH AMERICA.** Records, 1894-1910. Handwritten minutes book, 1894(founding meeting)-1910. 83 pp.
   With signatures of those attending 1st meeting.
A009. **BIERER, Bert W.** The veterinary sciences in South Carolina, 1887-1921. Typescript, 19 pp. §
   With reference to Univ SC and Clemson.
A010. **BIOGRAPHIES.** (31 items) British, American, French DVMs. §
   Short pieces from journals, many by C.H. Eby.
A011. **BOOKS AND BOOK COLLECTIONS.** (13 items). §
A012. **BRANDENBURG, T.O.; ROBINSON, J.W.** History of the North Dakota Veterinary Medical Association. 1962? Typescript (mimeo), 10 pp. §
   With list of presidents, 1903-1962.
A013. **BRITISH VETERINARY PROFESSION.** (8 items) §
   Includes veterinary surgeons' acts, 1881-1948.
A014. **BULLIS, K.L.** The Massachusetts Veterinary Association, 1884-[1959?]. Typescript, 16 pp. §
   Prepared for the 75th anniversary.
A015. **BUREAU OF ANIMAL INDUSTRY** (BAI). (5 items) §
   See also: Cattle Plague/Foot and Mouth Disease; Pistor, William P.
A016. **CADUCEUS.** (10 items) §
   Inappropriate origins of this quasimedical symbol.
A017. **CANADIAN VETERINARY PROFESSION.** (6 items) §
A018. **CARTY, James M.** (BVS) Practice account book, Morrisville, V[ermont], Jan 1917-Mar 1918. 60 pp. §

A019. **CATTLE PLAGUE/FOOT AND MOUTH DISEASE.** (4 items) §
See also: Bureau of Animal Industry; Pistor, William P.
A020. **COLTHAUS.** Dr. Colthaus' Universal Galen's Liniment. (Broadside), New York, ca 1870s. §
A021. **CROSS, Mary Ellen.** Original drawings, ca 1956. Historiated initial letters (mounted on cardboard) used in J.F. Smithcors: Evolution of the veterinary art, 1957. (27 items) §
A022. **CURES, Early.** (14 items, including photocopy of Cotton Tufts' article on horn distemper, 1735). §
A023. **DARLEY, Robert.** Manuscript receipt book. "Receipts of the art of Farriery and other objects useful to aney Perfect Groom." [Italy?], April 15, 1553. 42 pp.

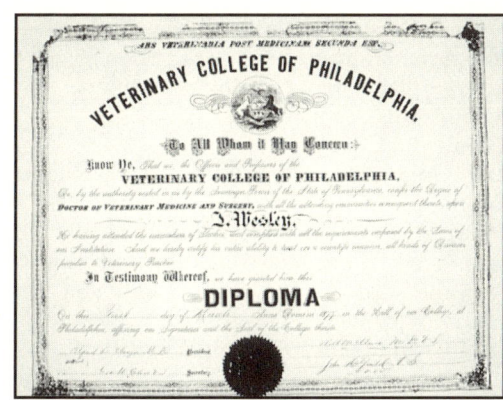

Veterinary college of Philadelphia: Diploma, 1877
(A024)

A024. **DIPLOMAS.** §
__ (a). Detroit Veterinary Dental College. December 3, 1907. With letter indicating this was by correspondence (!).
__ (b). Pennsylvania College of Veterinary Surgeons. June 13, 1881. A reputable diploma-granting body (not a school).
__ (c). Veterinary College of Philadelphia. March 1877. Has seal of Merchants' Veterinary College. (With "McClure's College" material. See main catalog entry 1344.) Was used to convict Robert McClure of forgery.
__ (d). Veterinary Science Association, London, Ontario, Canada. November 18, 1897. A correspondence school for farmers, run by the Detroit Veterinary Dental College.
A025. **DOGS.** Diseases and treatment, British. (6 items) §
A026. **EDUCATION AND RESEARCH.** (20 items) §
See also: Schools and Colleges.
A027. **EGYPTIAN VETERINARY MEDICINE.** (4 items) §
Includes photocopy of Papyrus of Kahun, ca 1800 BC.
A028. **FARRIERY AND HORSESHOEING.** (16 items) §
See also: Welch, Farrell F.

A029. **FOOD HYGIENE.** History of food control; history of meat inspection in the US. (2 items) Mimeo, ca 1945. 20 pp. §
   Syllabus for a course at College of Vet Med, Cornell.
A030. **GRAHAM, L(averne) P.** Papers, 1930s-1940s. (5 items) Laboratory workbooks (3) of a student at Ohio State University, ca 1940s. With W.F. Guard: Laboratory guide for operative veterinary surgery, 1936, 157 pp; and Course outline for general surgery, ca 1940s, 96 pp. §
A031. **HALL, A.V.** Therapeutics. Typescript and mimeo of course syllabus. San Francisco Veterinary College. 1890? 89 pp. §
A032. **HISTORY, General (Veterinary).** (11 items) §
   See also: Moule, Leon T.
A033. **HISTORY, Military.** See: Military, General (Veterinary); Military, World War I; Miller, Everett B.; Murnane, Thomas G.
A034. **HISTORY, Specialties.** (6 items) §
   Dermatology, ophthalmology, radiology, toxicology.
A035. **HOSPITALS, Animal.** (3 items) §
   See also: Schools and Colleges.
A036. **ILLUSTRATIONS.** (23 items, including "Great Moments in Veterinary Medicine," 6 color prints; 7 old prints.) §
A037. **MEMORABILIA.** Envelope postmarked Aug. 3, 1929 and addressed to H. Preston Hoskins, long-term secretary of AVMA when it was located in Detroit, purportedly in the hand of J.V. Lacroix, owner and editor of The North American Veterinarian. §
A038. **MICHIGAN CAPITOL VETERINARY MEDICAL ASSOCIATION.** Fee schedule, 1917. (Broadside) §
   Lists minimum prices "to be adhered to by our members."
A039. **MILITARY, General.** (Veterinary) (6 items) §
A040. **MILITARY, World War I.** Photographs of animal transport and care. (7 items) §
   See also: Ambulances, Animal.
A041. **MILLER, Everett B.** Papers, 1959-79. (9 items, 3-20 pp) §
   Includes veterinary military history, education, etc.
A042. **MOULE, Leon T.** History of veterinary medicine. Typescript (photocopy) of English translations from the French by Carl Olson and Rose Kastelic, ca. 1993. 613 pp. §
   See also: History, General (Veterinary).
A043. **MURNANE, Thomas G.** "Military heritage of veterinary medicine." Paper presented to Association of Military Surgeons of the United States, Nov. 29, 1977. Washington, DC. (photocopy) 18 pp. §
   See also: Military, General; Miller, Everett B.
A044. **MUSE, Raymond; FRYKMAN, George A.** Oral histories. Washington State University, Pullman, WA, 1973-79. (39 items). Tapes and transcripts of interviews with 39 DVMs, mainly from the Northwest.
A045. **MUSEUMS.** (8 items) §
A046. **OBSTETRICS AND REPRODUCTION.** (6 items) §

A047. **PATHOLOGY.** (6 items) §

A048. **PISTOR, W(illiam) P.** Papers, 1940s-1950s. Collection of documents (correspondence, BAI bulletins, etc.) almost all of which relate to the outbreak of foot-and-mouth disease in Mexico (ca 1946-). See also: Bureau of Animal Industry, Cattle Plague.

A049. **PORTRAITS.** Mostly of American veterinarians. (18 items) §

A050. **PUBLIC HEALTH.** (94 items) §

Includes "What the veterinary profession means to mankind," a series of 83 ads by Allied Labs appearing in Veterinary Medicine, 1940-46 (photocopies).

A051. **RABIES.** (15 items) §

Includes 10 reprints of articles by J. Theodorides (Paris).

A052. **RECEIPT BOOK.** Apparently the receipt book of an American veterinarian, in his hand. ca 1850s. 37 pp of entries. §

A053. **RECEIPT BOOK.** "Receipt book and horses." Autograph commonplace and receipt book. [England?] 1810-1815. Approximately 38 pp devoted to horses and receipts.

A054. **RELIGION AND MYTHOLOGY.** (4 items) §

A055. **REMINISCENCES.** A series of "reflections" by retired American veterinarians, from JAVMA, 1991-94. §

A056. **SCHOOLS AND COLLEGES.** (32 items, including 8 mounted photographs of University of Pennsylvania veterinary hospital, 1885; engraving of American Veterinary College, New York, "hospital department," from Harper's Weekly, March 12, 1881.) §

See also: Education and Research.

A057. **SMITHCORS, J(ames) F(rederick).** Papers, 1954-88. §

___ (a). The American veterinary profession. 1960. Typescript with reference citations in margins not included in the published work (catalog item 1344). Four loose-leaf notebooks. §

___ (b). Collected papers on veterinary history, 1954-1988. Reprints of 63 articles, etc, from 20 different veterinary and medical journals. Subjects include veterinary history, diseases, education, etc, with table of contents.

___ (c). Functional animal morphology, Parts I, II. School of Veterinary Medicine, Michigan State University, East Lansing, MI. 1949. Mimeo, 307 pp. Text for a 30-credit integrated course in veterinary anatomy, histology, embryology (first in US).

___ (d). Letters. (6 items, some with attachments), 1918-77. Subjects include veterinary schools, D.E. Salmon, Carlo Ruini, A. Liautard.

___ (e). Oral histories. AVMA meetings, 1959-60. (6 items) Cassette tapes of interviews with 29 prominent veterinarians.

___ (f). Sex, psyche, soma: a narrative account of medical word origins. Santa Barbara, CA. 1960. Unpublished typescript (photocopy). 284 pp. Presented by body systems, as in dissection.

___ (g). Veterinariana. 1959-75. A collection of short narratives related to veterinary history, animals, etc, from Modern Veterinary Practice, 1959-61. Bound with 100 selected MVP editorials, 1963-75. (photocopies). 130 pp.

A058. **SURGERY.** (7 items). §

A059. **UNITED STATES VETERINARY MEDICAL ASSOCIATION.** Minutes book (handwritten), 1863-98. Microfilm (35-mm). §

A060. **WASHBURN, E.A.** Papers, 1850-58. §

    ___ (a). Receipt book. Adrian, MI, ca 1850s. 40 pp.

    ___ (b). Receipt book (2), Adrian, MI, 1850-51. 100 pp; 1852-54. 85 pp.

    ___ (c). Autograph letter from George H. Dadd, Boston, MA, March 19, 1858, regarding Washburn's inquiry about veterinary books and "qualifying" to practice. 2 pp.

A061. **WELCH, Farrell F.** Receipt book for diseases in horses by an American farrier/blacksmith (?), in his hand. Southington, [CT?], June 6, 1879. 20 pp.

    See also: Farriery and Horseshoeing.

A062. **WOMEN VETERINARIANS.** (3 items) §

    See also: Association for Women Veterinarians.

Appendix Index

A

Account books, A018, A061
Advertising, Promotions, A001
Ambulances, A002, A040
American Animal Hospital Association, A003
American Veterinary College, A056
Anatomy, course syllabus, A057c
Animals, narratives, A057g; welfare, A006
ASPCA, Newburgh, NY, A004
Association of Veterinary Faculties, A008

B

Barker's "Komic" Picture Souvenir, A001
Bergh, Henry, A004b
Biographies, veterinarians, A010
Books, early, A011
Broadsides, A020, A038
Bureau of Animal Industry, A015, A048

C

Caduceus, A016
Colthaus, liniment, A020

D

Dadd, George H., A060
Detroit Veterinary Dental College, A024a
Diplomas, A024
Diseases: cattle, A019; cures, A022; dogs, A025; rabies, A051

E

Education, A026; schools, A024, A056, A057d
Egypt, veterinary medicine, A027
Etymology, medical/ veterinary, A057f
Evolution of the veterinary art, A021

F

Farriery, Horseshoeing, A028, A061
Food hygiene, A029
Foot-and-mouth disease, A019, A048

G

Graphics, A021, A036, A049, A056

H

History, military, A039, A040, A041, A043; general, A032, A042, A057bg; oral, A044, A057e; specialties, A034
Horn distemper, Cotton Tufts, A022
Hoskins, H. Preston, A037
Hospitals, animal, A035, A056

L

Liautard, A., A057d

M

Massachusetts, veterinary history, A014
Mexico, foot-and-mouth disease, A048
Michigan, fee schedule, A038
Miller, E.B., A041
Morris, Mark, A003cd
Murnane, T.G., A043
Museums, A045

N

North Dakota, veterinary history, A012

O

Obstetrics, Reproduction, A046
Ohio State University, workbooks, A030

P

Pathology, A047

Pennsylvania College of Veterinary Surgeons, A024b
Pennsylvania (Univ. of) Veterinary Hospital, A056
Public health, accomplishments, A050

R

Receipt books, A023, A052, A053, A060, A061
Religion, Mythology, A016, A054
Ruini, Carlo, A057d

S

Salmon, D.E., A049, A057d
South Carolina, veterinary history, A009
Surgery, A030, A058

T

Therapeutics, course syllabus, A031
Tufts, Cotton, horn distemper, A022

U

USMVA, minutes book, A059

V

Veterinarians, biographies, A010; portraits, A049; reminiscences, A044, A055, A057e
Veterinary College of Philadelphia, A024c
Veterinary history. See History, general; History, military; Miller, E.B.; Murnane, T.G.
Veterinary profession, American, A005; British, A013; Canadian, A017
Veterinary Science Association, A024d

W

Women veterinarians, A007, A062

Index

The catalog numbers listed in this index are the pertinent works for any given topic. Asterisks (*) indicate sources published before 1800, or those which deal mostly with this early period. The most important sources in regard to each topic are identified by boldface type. The collection includes works of all caliber, from the "good," even by today's standards, to the "bad," even at the time they were published. This index should prove useful in facilitating research into the many aspects of veterinary history, especially by persons unfamiliar with the older literature.

The following code letters identify the species indicated in the entries:

A avian
B bovine
C canine
D domestic animals
E Equine

F feline
H human
O ovine
P porcine
V veterinary

A

AAEP, 836
AAHA, 1540-43
Abildgaard, PC, 027
Abortion, B028, **130**, **318**, 350, 588, 613, 629, 743, 805, 861, 883, 1014, 1052, 1088, 1234, 1319. 1432, 1514, 1561, 1641, 1697; D1560; E1273, 1498
Actinomycosis, B001, 1369, 1370, 1499; D884, 1092, 1101, 1103
Age, 122*; B351, 964; C739, 784, 926; D739, **784**, **926**; E120, 136, 191*, 216, 298, 319, 351, 427, 498, 499, 503, 514, 520, 574, 611, 616, 670*, 698, 717, 812, 899, 940, 964, 975, 991*, 993, **1033**, 1121, 1170, 1272, 1273, 1384
Alabama VMA, 1539
Alfort Veterinary School, 1569
Almanacs, 014-025
Ambulances, 135
America, history, **V162**, 163, 164, **1344**, 1347; vet colleges, 209, 251
Anatomy, A829, 1402*; B147, 1080, 1697; C202, 466*, **489**, 1083; D283, 656, 683, **1312**; E129, **180**, 185*, 187*, 225, 248, 251, 356*, 379, **399**, 499,500, 587*, 694, 733, 749, 760, 763, 769, **868***, **932**, **1022**, 1079, 1121, **1166**, 1170, 1222*, **1255***, **1298**, 1310*, **1349***, **1393**, 1400*, 1402*, 1405*, 1617; F623, 874, 1083; H146, 254*, 466*, 596*, 1402*; O126, 1080, 1709; P1081; artistic, 117, 1295
Anesthesia, A829; B381; C746, 866, 1274; **D463**, **532**, 1034, 1152, 1548, 1559, 1563, 1565; E113, 647, 975; F746, 845, 874

Angell, GT, 036, 046
Angora cat, F800
Animal behavior, 755, F1031
Animal legislation, 050, 064, **071**, 078, 092, 106
Animal rights, 055, 069, **085, 091, 094**, 891, **894***
Animal welfare, 035-109
Animals in religion, 050, 067, 085, 1245, 1300; B359; E653; F782
Anthrax, **B**321, 327, 1173, 1369, 1432, 1517, 1697; C720; **D**523*, **526**, 560, 580, 724, 794, 883, 1045, 1092, 1103, 1249, 1279, 1501, 1512, 1550, 1560, 1607*, 1636; E652, 1237, 1671; O115, 170, **280**, **1151**, 1263; H720, 1025
Antibiotics, V1458
Antisepsis, H1040; V463, **559**, 570, 1373
Apoplexy, E1384
Appaloosa, E668
Arabian, 358; bibliography, 764
Artificial insemination, B785; C785; E785, 1563
Ascites, C1086
ASPCA, **035**, 082; also RSPCA
AVMA, 1346; proceedings, 1544-62
Azoturia, E861, 881, 1237, 1371, 1548, 1549

B

Bacteriology, H457, 1103; **V**219, 457, 667, 724, 1101
BAI, 775; annual reports, 1489-1531
Bang, B, 130
Behavior, 755; F1031
Bergh, H, 046, 082
Bighead, E110, 351, 408, 699, 700, 743, 993, 1257, 1321, **1384**, 1510
Biography,
    Abildgaard, PC, 027
    Angell, GT, 036, 046
    Bang, B, 130
    Bergh, H, 046, 082
    Dick, W, 432
    Evans, G, 1623
    Gamgee, J, 1443
    Hancock, R, 678
    Hobday, F, 745
    Horse doctor, 645
    Liautard, A, 1067

Marshall, B, 1406
McFadyean, J, 1157
Morris, M, 688
Osler, W, 378
Pearson, L, 1160
Poett, J, 950
Price, W, 1195
Smythe, R, 1348
Stubbs, G, 1403, 1406
Waddell, W, 1612
Welch, WH, 544
Young, W, 1727
Birds (caged), A171*, 1621, **1692**
Black veterinarians, 1610-13
Blacksmithing, 1228; history, 002, 1196, 1341
Bloat, **B**180, 321, **322**, 327, 343, 351, 381, 431, 503, 506, 588, 613, 743, 749, 812, 859, 875, 881, 964, 993, 1010, **1183**, 1367, 1370, 1432, 1697; O1709
Blood, C1364, 1554; **D**228, 580, 589, 1565; E113, 896, 1170, 1553; O1368; V518
Blood transfusion, B1565; C584; D231; E394, 1565
Bloodletting, **B**381, 393; C172, 335, 817; D351, 610, 929, **1181**, **1188***, 1432; E136, **138***, 176, 180, 192*, 198*, 253, **315***, 335, 379, 394, 413, **421***, 431, 500, 699, 717, **810**, 896, **901**, 978*, 982*, **1121**, 1351*, 1353*, 1361, **1439***, 1644, 1691*; O1709; V463, **1445**, 1536*
Bots, E192*, **253, 295**, 403, 431, 580, 589, 812, 813, 854, 982*, 1021, 1059*, 1060*, 1121, 1168, 1170, 1439*; O1709
Braxy, O634
Breaking, E120, **157**, 216, 309, 351, 414, 590, 613, **616**, 693, 717, 806, 808, 891, 901, **961, 964**, 975, 977, 1052, 1119, 1135, **1213**, 1226, 1241, 1384, 1392, 1426*, 1535, 1622*
Breeding, B124, 211, 318, 493, 805, **1148, 1477**, 1565; C152, 411, 714, 727, 1179, 1356*, 1452*, 1616; D419, 1046, 1173, 1513; E120, 124, 187*, **203***, **421***, 527, 607*, 717, 731, 806, 890, 977, 979*, 993, 1060*, 1119, **1148**, 1188*, 1264*, 1273, 1351*, 1353*, 1426*, 1537, 1565, 1607*, 1617, 1622*; O115, 124, 244, **1148**, 1209, 1263; P348, 710

Breeds, B124, 493, 888, 1052, 1697; C118*, 205, 235*, 411, 714, 896, **1430, 1616**; E124, 159*, **178**,249, 498, 806, 1052, **1537**; O126, 244, 888, 947, 1095, 1435, **1531**, 1709; P124, 347, 888, 1708

Britain, 630, 1328*, 1345*, 1563, 1593

Broken wind, E**143***, 171*, 218, 321, 500, 560, 603*, 653, 657*, 695, 733, 854, 901, 982*, 991*, 1004, 1132, **1168**, 1170, 1222*, 1237, 1353*

Bronchitis, B613

Brucellosis, goats, 1514

Bull terrier, C456, 612

Bull worship, B359

C

Calculi, C730, 746; D580, 875, 1681; E120; F746, 845

California, 111; vet coll, 803

Calving; see Parturition

Canada, 134, 1066

Canary, A1621, **1692**

Canker, C1003, 1086, 1364, 1698; F800, 1664

Castration, A829, **863**, 1660; B1100, 1367; C746,**863**, 922; D112*, **863**, 922, 1036, **1181**, 1637; E120, 138*, 210*, 238, 365, **394**, 699, 749, 891, 993, 1052, 1170, 1273, 1324, 1466, 1652; F746, 845, **863**; O1100, 1368; P155, 372, 1708; V463

Catalogs, books, 255, 273, 274; drugs, 262, 264, 266, 267, 270, 272; horseshoes, 269; instruments, 256, 258, 260, 263, 265, 268, 275

Cataract, E252, 356*, **1168**, 1536*

Catarrh, B812, 1546; C1105; D560, 880; E695, 733, 894*, 951, 1702

Cattle plague, 128, 1060; history, **1661**; see also Rinderpest

Cattle trade, 631, 632, 1495, 1496

Cautery, E231; V463, 929; see also Firing

Chicago VMA, 490

Choke, B180, 389; E1006, 1371

Chorea, C1086, 1178, 1364

Circulation, **686***; E460; H154*

Coach horses, E1127*

Colic, B180, 322, 381, 812; D560, 1279, 1563; E110, 120, 138*, 192*, **236**, 253, 300, 315*, 321, 350, 351, 365, 498, 520,
603*, 652, 695, 717, 733, **743**, 875, 881, 896, 901, 940, 961, 964, 1004. 1021, 1052, 1121, 1168, 1170, **1217**, **1268***, 1351*, 1353*, 1432, 1651, 1654, 1681

Conformation, E120, 187*, 248, 293, 343, 514, 520, 553, 607*, **624, 702,** 731, 766, **899,** 1059*, 1229, 1268*, 1351*, 1689, 1694

Contagion, E521; **V1536***

Cornell Univ, 917, 918, 1091, 1093, 1570

Cornstalk disease, B**1090**, 1508

Cough, E350

Cowpox, B028, **206,** 217, 321, 322, 345, **376,** 580, 725, 1111, 1162, 1367, 1624

Cruelty, 052, 053, 054, **089**; see also Animal welfare

Cryptorchidectomy, E238

Cysticercosis, history, P155

Cystitis, C214, 727, 1274; F214

D

Denmark-Russia, history, 823

Dehorning, B749, 944

Dentistry, CD739; E319, 321, 929, **1033**, 1545

Diabetes, C214; E356*, 652, 1237; F214

Diarrhea, B322, 351, 503, 805, 812, 1369, 1641, 1697; C172, 1003, 1086, 1176; D1279; E125, 335, 1168, 1170, **1237**, 1432; O351, 381; P155

Dick, W, 432

Dictionaries, 433-455; E413; V379, 399, 513; sporting, 1428

Diphtheria, C727

Disease reporting, 029

Diseases, A124, 362, 1270, **1621**, 1692; B277* 402, 424*, 1248, 1447*; C417, 418, 1454*; D011, 012, 205, 484*, 791*; E011, 124. 402, 424* 770*, 868*, 1207*, 1248, 1296*, 1311*, 1416*, 1447*, 1687*, 1691*; F172, 418, 874; H1397*; O124, 402, 1454*; P124, 351, 381, 1708; rabbit, 971, 1275

Disinfection, E1013; V410, 559, 853, 1331, 1548, 1550

Distemper, C028, 172, 176, 178, 184, 205, 214, 335, 351, 381, 415, 523*, **526,** 560, 584, 714, 727, **743, 817, 844,** 883, 901, 993, 1003, 1059*, 1063, 1086, 1088, 1092, 1105, 1173, 1176, 1178, 1272,

1274, **1297**, 1317, 1425*, 1430, 1550, 1616, **1698**; E157, 218, 253, 951, 1652; F214, 344, 726, **743**, 800, 845, 1275, 1664

Docking, E052, 058, 099, 138*, 180, 198*, 253, 394, 499, 500, 717, 806, 901, 993, 1036, 1257, 1652, 1702

Dog fighting, C612

Dogs, bibliography, 783; history, 118*, 1327, 1538, 1698

Dourine, E883, 1045, 1092, 1503, 1559, 1563, 1671

Draft animals, 1702

Dystocia, B150, **467**, 1162, 1173; C746; D534, 875; E1273; F746; O1149

E

Ear cropping, C052, 1698

Eclampsia, C727

Eczema, C1176, 1178

Edinburgh Vet Coll, 201, 1577

Education, V166, **180**, **221***, 251, **252**, 311, 381, 403, 1039, 1153, **1183**, 1197, **1259**, **1268***, 1289, 1544, 1546, 1553, 1556, 1562, **1661**

Elephants, 485

Emblems, V824

Embryology, A495; E494; H254*

Encephalitis, D882; E610, 1552, 1563

Enteritis, C214, 730, 1364, 1698; D795, 881; E204, 403, 695, 743, 1168, 1170, 1237; F214, 726, 845, 1275; P840, 1708

Epidemiology, V1291

Epilepsy, C1086, 1106; D882; E1222*

Epizootics, D1045; V163, 164, 775

Equitation; see Riding

Ergotism, B1111, **1483**

Erysipelas, P560

Ethics, V1020

Euthanasia, E125

Evans, G, 1623

Evolution, 755; B959; E702, 777, 1307, 1449

Exercise, E315*, 520, 646, 732, 1426*

Eye, C172, 214; D882, 1534; E896, 899, 901, 993, 1170, 1222*; F214; H1150, 1417; V1129, **1299**

F

Falconry, 160*, 178, 289*

Farcy, E253

Farming books, bibliography, 571, 572

Feeding, **A938**; B1475, 1506, **1515**; C172, 176, **938**. **1179**; D853, **938**, 1510; E180, **315***, 498, **607***, 732, 978*, 979*, 1132, 1145, 1379

Fertility; see Reproduction

Fever, B1697; C1615; D880; E138*, 143*, 329*, 403, 421*, 498, 499, 500, 503, 506, 603*, 731, 854, 894*, 982*, 1052, **1059***, 1060*, **1168**, 1170, 1222*, 1309*, 1317, 1644; H1258; V1445

Firing, E136, 138*, 180, 221*, 329*, **421***, 940, 1036, **1168**, 1360, 1432, 1439*, **1536***, 1563, 1652, 1702

First aid, CF920

Fistula, E365, 500, 733, 809, 810, 929, 977, 1006, 1027, **1032**, 1036, 1121, 1168, 1222*, 1544

Fog fever, B322, 854, 901

Folk medicine, B802; H802, 1185

Foot, B1367; E120, 124, **136**, 138*, **180**, 198*, 243, 248, **291**, 313*, 329*, 343, 351, **353***, **354**, 365, 403, 413, 431, 462, 476, **482**, 498, 499, 500, 503, 514, 520, 527, 528, **557***, 647, 657*, **666**, 671*, 689, 717, 731, 789, 869*, 870*, 899, 955, **961**, 982*, 991*, 1036, **1047**, 1069, 1159, **1186**, **1221**, **1232**, **1265**, 1268*, 1351*, **1360**, 1421*, 1429*, 1439*, 1536*, 1651, 1696*, 1702; bibliography, 1186

Foot-and-mouth disease, B032, 327, **526**, 580, 861, 1092, 1190, 1369, **1480**, 1506, 1511, 1517; D1681; O115; P840

Footrot, B506, 812, 854; O170, 322, 327, 343, 345, **526**, 812, 854, 940, 942, 964, 1095, 1209, 1263, 1368, 1378, 1432, 1445, 1709

Founder, B810; E176, 221*, 226, 286, **313***, 351, 356*, 403, 514, 671*, 695, 706, 809, 861, 993, 1014, 1121, 1168, 1268*, 1432, **1536***

Fowl cholera, 762, 912, 1470, 1480, **1481**, 1482

Foxes, 009

Fractures, C172, 214, 584, 866, 1698; D365, 1072, **1181**; E120, 568, 699, 1014, 1168, 1317, 1536*; F214; H1030, 1293; V532, 929

Freemartin, B351

G

Gait, E120, 178, **624**, 702, **896, 899**, 978*, 1229, **1389**, 1689
Game fowl, 362
Gamgee, J, 1443
Gapeworms, A1483
Gastritis, C1003; D881; E743, 1006; F726
Genetics, D419, 1046; E646, 698, **1172**
Genital disease, D1665; see also Dourine
Germany, history, 850
Gid, O244, 321, 377, 560, 613, 812, 1014, 1368, 1709
Giessen Vet Coll, 1284
Glanders, E120, 125, 136, **138***, 157, **180**, 191, 192*, 198*, 22l*, 253, 315*, 335, 343, 351, 365, 394, 403, 408, 413, 421*, 431, 500, 503, 514, 520, **526**, 560, 588, 603*, 652, 706, 724, 731, 733, 743, 794, **808**, 810, 812, 869*, 870*, 883, 894*, 896, 964, 975, 982*, 991*, 993, 1004, 1010, 1014, 1021, 1045, 1052, 1059*, 1088, 1092, 1101, 1159, **1168**, 1192, 1222*, 1264*, **1268***, **1353***, 1439*, **1478**, 1487, **1493**, 1513, 1552, 1554, 1555, 1557, 1560, 1562, **1606**, 1644, **1651**, 1702; H883, 1025
Gleet, E695
Goats, **1504**, 1505, 1514
Guide dogs, history, C361*

H

Hancock, R, 678
Haw, E1183
Hawks, 160*, 979*, 1161; see also Falconry
Heart, B685; C1106; D311, 580, 794, 880; E120, 652; H121
Heaves, E125, 351, 685, 749, 880, 1014
Hemorrhage, D794; E869*, 870*
Hen fever, 229
Heredity, E421*, 1273; see also Genetics
Hernia, B327, 389, 1111; C214, 558, 746, 1105; D1036, 1072, **1181**, 1563, 1681; E120, 138*, 516, 1014, **1168**; F214, 746; P372, 861; V929
Histology, D486; H752, 1632; V683
History; see also Vet Assn; Vet Coll
America, 162-4, 166, 1039, 1344, 1347

Bureau Anim Industry (BAI), 775
Blacksmithing, 002, 1196, 1341
Britain, 630, 1328*, 1345*, 1563, 1593
California, 111
Canada, 134, 1066
Cattle plague, 1661
Danish-Russian, 823
Dogs, 118*, 783, 1327, 1538, 1698
Ethics, 1020
Guide dogs, 361
Hog cholera, 169, **1471**, **1489**
Horse, 159, 292, 429
Humane movement, 080, 100
Illinois, 207
Indiana, 1391
Iowa, 1113
Japan, 1118
Kansas, 481
Maryland, 1442
Medical illustration, 722
Medicine, 591, 1040
Michigan, 1097
Military, 548, 1039, 1056, 1330*
Mississippi, 936
Nebraska, 916, 1115
New Jersey, 1441
New York, 919
North Carolina, 1094
Ontario, 492
Ophthalmology, 970
Pennsylvania, 1399, 1440
Plagues, 163, **523***
Publications, 1584-94
Rabies, 530
Research, 1289, 1450
Riding, 288
Rinderpest, 189, 577
Scabies, 565
Shoeing, 299, **524***, 1196
Smallpox, 597
SPCA, 042, 051
Sweden, 677
Tennessee, 847
Turkey, 491
Vet med (general), 166, **180***, 252, 290*, 403, 821*, 908*, 909*, 1328, 1345, 1544, 1557, 1614*, 1661
Virginia, 511
Hobday, F, 745

140 *Five Centuries of Veterinary Medicine*

Hog cholera, 164, 165, **169**, 196*, 203*, 226, 318, 321, **347**, 372, 389, 554, 588, 633, 743, 762, **840**, 861, 883, 940, 942, 952, 1137, 1151, 1432, **1477, 1479, 1489, 1491**, 1492, 1493, 1498, 1502, 1507, 1511, 1544, 1560; history, **1471, 1489**
Hollow horn; see Hornail
Homeopathy, **C1086**; **D**350, 816, 942, **1085**; **E**717, **1087**; **V**664, **756**, 759, 786, 797, **1088, 1260, 1279**
Hornail, **B**028, 381, 393, 809, 810, 813, 1429*, **1432**, 1445
Horse, bibliography, 659; history, 159*, 292, 429
Horse taming; see Breaking
Horsemanship; see Riding
Horsepox, **E**120, **526**, 1237
Human-animal bond, 731, 822, 896
Humane movement, 035-109; **E**221*, 958, 1135; **V**1173; see also Animal welfare
Humane treatment, **B**381; **E**225, 394, 890
Hunting, **C**152, 160*, **178**, 205, 281*, 415, 776, 814*, 817, 862, 896, 901, 980*, 1428, 1430, 1452*; **E**891, 1131, 1226, 1428
Husbandry, Roman, **D**276*, 792*, 793*, 1607*
Hygiene, **V**166, **315***, 410, 421*, 483, **526**, 695, **853**, 1302, **1331, 1536***
Hysteria, **E**403

I

Illinois, 207
Illustration, medical, 722, 1252*
Immunization, **V**570; see also Vaccination
Indian, American, **E**1244, 1609; **H**1609
Indiana, 1391, 1564, 1565
Indigestion, **B**1369; **C**558, 1178; **D**1456; **E**120, 125, 1547
Infectious anemia, **E**794, 1092, 1558, 1636
Inflammation, **B**180, 327, 381, 393, 812, 901, 1088; **D**880, 1324; **E**143*, 225, 431, 499, 520, 652, **697**, 706, 732, 858, 993, 1021, 1159, **1168**, 1241, **1619**, 1651; **O**345; **V**610
Influenza, **E**252, 321, 394, 403, 521, 523*, **526**, 560, 588, 589, 647, 698, 743, 756, 794, 883, 940, 951, 1006, 1021, 1045, 1088, 1237, 1324, 1371, **1476**, 1636, 1671
Iodine therapy, **V**1373
Iowa, 1113; vet college, 1144, 1363

J

Japan, 1118
Jaundice, **C**214, 727, 1176; **D**881; **E**403, 854, 982*, 1222*; **F**214
Joints, **B**1100; **C**1105; **E**120, 136, 568, 1010, **1168**, 1221
Jurisprudence, American, **E**679, **V**709; British, **E**1375; **V**220, 638, 640, 778, 1331; French, 360, 935; German, **V**161, 1302

K

Kansas, 481; Kansas City VC, 1573

L

Lameness, **E**124, 138*, 216, 221*, 313*, 315*, 321, 394, 646, 756, **864**, 891, 896, 901, **928**, 954, 961, 964, 1006, 1010, 1084, **1132**, 1140*, **1168, 1232**, 1264*, 1351*, 1360, 1554, 1562, 1563, 1635, 1654, **1695**; **P**155
Laminitis, **E**180, 365, 516, 522, 1006, 1085, 1168, **1221**, 1232, 1324, 1360
Lampas, **E**157
Law; see Jurisprudence
Liautard, A, 1067
Ligation, 939
Locoism, **BEO**989, **B**1010
London vet college, 364, 627, 1199, 1575*
Longhorns, **B**460
Louping ill, **O**634
Lung plague; see Pleuropneumonia
Lymphangitis, **E**120

M

Mad itch, **B**351
Malleus, **V1536***
Mange, **B**813, 1367, 1506, 1549, 1553, 1555; **C**152, 172, 335, 730, 817, 896, 901, 1003, 1106, 1176, 1178, 1274, 1430, 1616; **D**365, **526**, 560, 580, 795, 1100, 1188*, 1456, 1607*; **E**192*, 321, 421*, 695, 1004, 1045, 1168, 1170, 1421*, 1431, 1439*, 1549; **F**726, 800, 845; **O**203*, 1014, 1052; **P**1708; see also Scab

Markham, G, bibliography, 1193
Marshall, B, 1406
Maryland, 1442
Mastitis, **B008**, 321, 343, 351, 365, 503, 546, 685, 743, 810, 1014, 1027, 1100, 1367, 1370, 1432, 1563; D534; E809; F726; O1368
Materia medica, B1367; E120, **136**, **143***, 188*, 413, 1087, 1353*, 1651, 1702; H218, **459***, 477*, **1188***, 1436, **1690**; O115, 1209; V131, 149, 212, **381**, **470**, 517, 566, **599**, 613, 649, 681, 690, 742, 744, 756, **1053**, **1098**, 1162, **1201**, 1418, 1453, 1459, **1682**
McFadyean, J, 1157
Meat inspection, B582; V**483**, 578, 724, **1142**, 1308, 1387, 1468, 1511, 1513, 1514, 1547, 1548, 1550, 1563
Medication, C1615; E176, 421*, 499, 682, 1421*; H497; P155; V681
Medicine, bibliography, 663; history, 591, 1040
Medieval hippiatry, bibliography, 1192*
Meningitis, C1106; D560, 795; E286, 1501, 1510, 1563
Mercurialization, V1445
Metritis, B006; C1106, 1178; D743; F726
Michigan, 1097; vet college, 1576
Microscopy, 752
Military VM, E026, 250, 374, 408, 1231, 1462; equitation, 1461, 1464, 1465; history, 548, 1039, 1056, 1330; Vet Corps, 1466
Milk fever, B008, 321, **322**, 343, 350, 365, 389, 561, 685, 749, 756, 861, 882, 964, 1010, 1085, 1319, 1370, 1432, 1445, 1456, 1548, 1551, 1697
Milk hygiene, B008, 724, 1128, 1355, 1476, 1504, 1512, 1548, 1556, 1557, 1558, 1559
Milk sickness, B008, 351, 389, 393, 724, 1185, 1432; D883; H381, 1185
Milk yield, B318, 546, 662, **705**, 1475, 1509
Mississippi, 936
Missouri, 661; vet college, 661
Morris, Mark, 688
Mortality, E740

Mules, 011, 210*, 374, 527, 717, **993**, 1060*, 1148, 1173, **1230**, 1231, 1257, 1321, 1499, 1510
Murrain, B203*, 322, 343, 351, 506, 810, 812, 901, 993, 1253*, 1697; O711*
Muscles, C466*; D1315; E294, 1170; H208*, 466*, 1198*; V518
Museums, Nebraska, 1115; Sweden, 1114
Mythology, E781; F409, 782, 1031

N

Nasal gleet, E695
Natural history, 112*, 122*, 1188*, 1245
Navel ill, E861
Nebraska, 916, 1115
Necropsy, C1063; D226, **375**; V426, 610
Negligence, E679; see also Jurisprudence
Neonatal disease, D534, 1669; E861
Neoplasms; see Tumors
Neurotomy, E120, 403, 1004, 1036, 1052, **1163**, **1168**, 1170, 1360, 1554, 1654, 1702
New Jersey, 1441
New York, 919, 1568
New York City VMA, 1567
North Carolina, 1094
Nursing, H1130
Nutrition, A938; C938; D355, 938

O

Obstetrics, B211; C746, 1274; D534, 1010; E113, 1434; F746; H1254*; V554, 1667, **1669**
Ohio, 357; vet college, 1282
Ontario, 492; vet college, 595
Ophthalmia, C1086; E113, 125, 136, 138*, 180, 286, 321, 365, 580, 603*, 882, 1004, **1168**, 1562, 1644
Ophthalmology, H1150, 1417; V1129, **1299**, 1534; history, V970
Osteomalacia, B389
Osteoporosis, E882, 1546
Ostrich, 1621
Otitis, C1176, 1178
Oxen, 343, 462, 894*

P

Pain, 076
Parasites, A829, 916, 1161, 1270, 1620; B028, 124, 180, 321, 327, 1367, **1484**,

1504, 1512, 1514, 1517; C214, 584, 727, 964, 1063, 1086, 1105, 1176, 1179, 1364; D242, 743, **795, 826,** 875, **884,** 1010, 1139, 1249, 1387, 1456, **1460,** 1505, 1636, 1671; **E246,** 647, 652, 731; F214, 1275; O028, 115, 124, 126, 327, **377, 964,** 1263, 1504, 1511, 1552; P155, 347, 372, 840, 964, 1388; V346, **672, 1125;** bibliography, V1473

Parturition, B150, 322, 327, 343, 351, 365, 389, 393, 467, 506, 685, 749, 805, 813, 854, 859, 901, 964, 1014, 1027, 1052, 1253*, 1319, 1367, 1377, 1445, 1517, 1641; C714, 727, **1003,** 1063, 1179, 1364, 1698; **D534;** E120, 365, 749, 1324, 1377, 1434; H1254*; O115, **1149,** 1377, 1392, 1709; P155

Pathology, C152; E286; H1632; **V311,** 426, **841,** 849, **851,** 1035, **1092,** 1249, 1256, 1671; history, 1276, 1390

Pearson, L, 1160

Pennsylvania, 1399, 1440; vet college, 1580

Percheron, 469, 1019

Pharmacology, E188*; V665, 742, **1053**

Pharmacopoeia, B650; E143*, 185*, 302, 651, 993, 1651; H477*, 1436, 1690; V149, **335, 470,** 566, **570, 599,** 649, 690, **1053, 1098,** 1162, 1418, **1453**

Phlebitis, E977, 1006, 1168

Physiology, 245, 1245; E129, 356*, 379, 1170; H370, 479, 848; **V311,** 355, 518, 683, 1156, **1333, 1342**

Plague, B203*; D163, **523*; V1536*;** see also Cattle Plague

Piroplasmosis, D794; see also Texas fever

Pleuropneumonia, B318, 321, 327, **389,** 393, 431, 523*, **526,** 580, 613, 635, 743, 756, **805, 879,** 883, 944, 1014, 1085, 1154, 1173, 1367, 1369, 1469, **1470,** 1474, **1479, 1480,** 1483, **1484,** 1485, 1486, **1490,** 1491, 1493, 1495, 1496, 1497, 1517, 1544, 1662, 1671

Pneumonia, B322, 880, 1500; C1176, 1274; D560, 795, 1279, 1546, 1636; E125, 180, 321, 394, 403, 652, 743, 880, 1006, **1168,** 1324, 1371, 1560; F344; P155, 840

Poett, J, 950

Poisonous plants, 126, 873, **1146**

Poisons, B989, 1367, 1517; C1364; D351, 853, 881, 1100, 1279, 1456, 1551; E113, 120, 647, 652, 699, 989, 1183, 1371, 1384; F344, 845; H459*, 1138; O126, 989, 1368; P155; V560, **855**

Poll evil, E120, 157, 329*, 365, 394, 500, 503, 671*, 733, 812, 858, 896, 921, 929, 977, 982*, 993, 1004, 1006, 1027, **1032,** 1036, 1168, 1222*, 1317, 1536*

Poultry, 007*, 011, 229, 351, 515, 588, 756, 791*, 1161, 1270, 1509

Pox, D525, 743, 794, 883; O1209

Predators, A1161

Preventive medicine, E695; V327, 526, 853, 1291

Price, W, 1195

Psychology, D937

Public health, B1340; E1013; H708, 1128, **1251,** 1278, **1290,** 1303, 1340; **V166, 526,** 544, 578, 582, **1142, 1197, 1251,** 1278, **1290,** 1301, 1303, 1387, 1557, 1565, 1661

Pulse, E125, 136, 253, 315*, **499,** 503, 520, 695, 732

Purchase, E157, 167, 191*, 196*, 198*, 218, 221*, 253, 343, 427, 499, 500, 503, 549, 616, 679, 717, **766,** 809, 810, 812, 854, 891, 894*, 975, **977,** 1226, 1375, 1429*, 1431, 1654; V935

Purgation, C817; D1545; E138*, 180, 192*. 198*, 221*, 225, 253, **315*,** 335, 421*, 431, 500, 732, 894*, 982*, 1060*, 1132, 1317, 1353*, 1361, 1421*, 1431, **1439***

Purpura, B883; E516, 883, 1237, 1324, 1371

Q

Quackery, 005*, 888; E282, 319, 657*, 872, 1135, 1535; H1180

R

Rabbit diseases, 971, 1275

Rabies, B203*, 351, 1090; C028, 112*, **133, 172,** 176, 214, 234, 335, 351, 381, 415, 431, 580, **622, 714,** 724, 727, 756, **817,** 896, 901, 993, 1003, 1105, 1176, 1188*, 1274, 1317, **1356*,** 1364, **1415,** 1430. **1437, 1452*,** 1500, 1512, 1549, 1630, **1631,** 1652, **1698;** D365, 523*,

526, 530, 560, 724, 743, 794, 883, 1040, 1045, 1279. 1504, 1510, 1546, 1548, 1636, 1671; E143*, 731, 756, 1702; F214, 726, 845; H128, **133, 530, 622,** 833, 1025, 1040, **1303, 1415,** 1512, 1555, 1630, **1631;** O244, 1209, 1263; P155, 1708; history, D530

Racehorses, 306, 1229, 1318

Racing, E178, 205, 288*, 414, 616, 731, 780, 891, 901, 940, 975, 978*, 993, 1019, 1131, 1173, 1257, 1426*, 1617

Radiology, C746, **846, 1286;** D231; E482; F746, **846**

Red water, B180, 322, 327, 389, 812, 854, 901, 1641

Remount, regulations, E1465

Reproduction, **686;** B006, 785, 1562; C172, 1615; D112*, 335, 534, **990,** 1339, 1665; E210*, 785, 1273; O1709

Research, 1289, 1450

Restraint, B964; E120, 216, 296, 305, 480, 1535; V463, **532,** 929, 1034, **1638**

Rheumatism, B1100; D882

Riding, E158*, 171*, 288*, 480, 552. **556,** 575*, **590,** 607*, 717, 890, 894*, 896, 979*, 1052, 1164*, **1226,** 1309*, 1351*, 1416*, 1438*, 1461, 1464, 1680; bibliography, 552, 1634; history, 288*

Rinderpest, **B031,** 032, 186*, **189,** 389, 523*, **526,** 577, **582,** 613, 636, 1014, 1045, 1052, 1173, 1367, 1469, **1475, 1479,** 1487, 1517, 1671; history, 189, 577; see also Cattle plague

Roaring, E113, 120, **232,** 431, **531,** 560, 580, 647, 653, 695, 699, 743, 880, 929, 958, 1004, 1006, 1021, 1036, **1132,** 1168, **1170,** 1318, **1353*,** 1547, 1555, 1556, 1560, 1563, 1646, 1654, 1702

Roman husbandry, D276*, 792*, 793*

Rot (liver flukes), O170, 203*, 244, 321, 322, 343, 351, 377, 381, 901, 993, 1014, 1052, 1095, 1209, 1263, 1429*, 1432, **1709**

Rowelling, E1426*

RSPCA, 042, 051, 063, 100; see also ASPCA

S

Scab, O196*, 322, 345, 351, 377, 580, 812, 901, 1096, 1188*, 1209, 1263, 1368, 1378, 1429*, 1431, 1501, 1504, 1506, 1607*, 1709; see also Mange

Scabies, H565

Scarletina, D1279; E394, 695, 1237

Septicemia, D794, 1636

Sheep pox, 115, 327, **345, 526,** 589, **1052,** 1209, **1306**

Shipping fever, B1517, 1551, 1557

Shock, V1034

Shoeing, **B462;** E120, 136, 138*, 216, 218, 248, **251,** 252, **253,** 291, 309, **313*,** 353*, 354, 408, 414, **462,** 476, 498, 520, **522, 524*, 528,** 557*, 590, 616, 689, 789, 868*, 869*, **870*,** 891, **894*,** 896, 901, **955, 961, 964,** 1047, 1059*, 1112, 1140* 1164*, 1196, **1225,** 1241, 1264*, **1265, 1268*,** 1351*, **1353*,** 1426*, 1545, 1617, 1689, 1702; history, **299, 524*,** 1196

Slaughter, 057, 061, 078, 081, 1308

Smallpox, **H206,** 217, **376,** 458*, 525, 704, 725, 1292, 1624, 1693; history, 597

Smythe, R, 1348

Snakebite, C817; D884

Soundness, E120, 136, 403, 427, 646, **692, 698,** 778, 958, 1052, **1172,** 1689

Spanish conquest, E625

Spanish VM, bibliography, 949

Spasm, E192*

Spavin, E403, 498, 1006, 1614, 1644

Spaying, B238, 381, 393, 613, 805, 1563; C172, 214, 558, **727,** 746, **863, 922,** 1274, **1452*;** D863, **922,** 1036, **1181, 1637;** E238, 1560; F214, 746, **863;** O1709; P372, 381, 901; V463

Sprains, E120, 138*, 180, 313*, 699

Staggers, E138*, 157, 191, 192*, 218, 329*, 394, 421*, 580, **657*,** 894*, 896, 977, 982*, 1004, 1170, 1384, 1654

Sterility, **B006,** 685; CD785; see also Reproduction

Strangles, E138*, 191*, 192*, 253, 321, 335, 356*, 403, 457, 603*, 743, 812, 1004, 1121, 1222*, 1237, 1279, 1324, 1353*, 1439*, 1536*, 1636; P1708

State boards, V837

Stomach tube, B1183, **1253***

Stubbs, G, 1403, 1406

Sulfonamides, V1458

Surgery, A1621; B723; C234, 584, 746, 866, **1274**; D719, 1559; E230, 297, **568**, 723, 1617; F746; H168, 215*; V148, **463, 532, 929, 1034, 1036, 1072**, 1553, 1554, 1667, **1677**; instruments, 156*, 1294*
Surra, B1512; E1505
Swamp fever; see Infectious anemia
Sweden, 677, 1114
Sweeny, E408
Swine fever; see Hog cholera
Swine plague, 372, 840, 944, 1469, **1470, 1474, 1478, 1479, 1480,** 1481, **1484, 1487, 1490,** 1491, 1492, 1496, 1498, 1499, 1502

T

Tapeworm, A1508; P155, 1708
Teat surgery, B008
Teeth, B389, 805; C739, 784; D580, 739, 784, 926; E298, **319,** 350, 574, 588, **611, 624,** 685, 698, 975, 1033, 1052, 1168, 1170, 1384, 1689
Temperament, E480, 982*
Tennessee, 847
Tetanus, B393; D365, 560, 580, 610, 724, 794, 883, 1103, 1548, 1636; E113, 120, 125, 204, 218; 226, 253, 321, 350, 394, **403,** 516, 603*, **653,** 695, **697,** 706, 896, 901, 975, 977, 1004, 1006, 1014, 1052, 1088, **1168,** 1170, 1237, 1324, 1371, 1429*, 1536*, **1630,** 1702; H1025
Texas, vet college, 1285
Texas fever, B164, 279, 613, **628,** 745, 756, 883, 942, 1010, 1014, 1111, 1369, 1432, 1469, 1470, **1480,** 1481, 1483, **1484, 1485,** 1486, **1490,** 1495, 1497, 1498, **1499,** 1502, 1503, **1504,** 1509, 1510, 1513, 1517, 1544, 1547, 1550, 1551, 1557, 1636, 1681
Therapeutics, D488; V131, **570,** 649, 690, 742, 867, **1053, 1203,** 1418, 1459, **1682**
Thermometry, 116
Toxicology, V855, **873,** 1203
Training, C184, 414, 714, 1241, 1663; D937; E119, 203*, **616,** 808, 961, 1112, 1194, 1241, 1622*, 1663
Transport, B090
Trembles; see Milk sickness
Trichinosis, P1388

Tuberculosis, A1545, 1552; B032, **033,** 124, 130, 226, **423, 526,** 724, 820, **856,** 887, 1100, 1111, **1116,** 1128, 1216, 1234, **1278, 1301,** 1340, 1367, 1369, 1370, 1488, **1494,** 1498, 1502, 1505-8, 1511, 1513, 1517, 1548, 1550, 1552-4, 1556, 1558, 1559; C234; D560, 641-4, **883,** 1084, 1092, 1101, 1103, **1142,** 1500, 1504, 1510, 1549, 1636; E403; F845, 874, 1275, 1664; H378, 641-4, **856,** 1025, **1116,** 1139, 1216, **1278;** P1556
Tumors, A829, 1026; B1517; C214, **558,** 584, 1105; D1249, 1552, 1556; E568, 652; F214, 1664; **V512**
Turin, vet college, 1582
Turkey, 491
Turkish bath, DH1532

U

Udder, B008; see also Mastitis
Urine, C1106; D589; E652, 1168, 1560; V518
USCVS, 1583
USDA, 1469-1531
USVMA; see AVMA
Uterine prolapse, E238

V

Veterinary associations,
    AAEP, 836
    AAHA, 1540-43
    Alabama, 1539
    AVMA, 1346, 1544-62
    British, 1563
    Chicago, 490
    Indiana, 1564-65
    Iowa, 1566
    New York, 1568
    New York City, 1567
    Ohio, 357
    Ontario, 492
    Pathology, 1390
    Virginia, 511
Veterinary colleges,
    Alfort, 1569
    California, 803
    Cornell, 917-8, 1091, 1093
    Edinburgh, 201, 1577
    Giessen, 1284

Index   145

Iowa, 1144, 1363
Kansas City, 1573
London, 364, 627, 1199, 1575
Michigan, 1576
Missouri, 661
Ohio, 1282
Ontario, 595
Pennsylvania, 1580
Texas, 1285
Turin, 1582
USA, 209, 251
USCVS, 1583
Vienna, 1283
Washington, 857
World, 908
Veterinary Corps, 1466, 1467; see also Military VM
Veterinary hygiene; see Hygiene
Veterinary periodicals, American, 1595-98, 1600, 1601, 1605; British, 1599, 1602-04; Veterinary history, 1584-94
Vienna, vet college, 1283
Vices, E303, 765, 1052, 1119, 1194
Vivisection, 036, 038, **039**, 043, 045, 047, **056**, 070, **072-075**, 079, 083, 086, **089**, 093, 095, 102-109; see also Animal welfare
Volvulus, D795
Vomiting, D580

W

Waddell, W, 1612
Warranty, **E679**, 698, **778**, 891, 958, 1375; V935
Washington, vet college, 857
Welch, WH, 554
Witchcraft, D754, 1155; E545, 781; F409; H754, 1180
Wolf (tail), B196*, 203*, 389, 1431; E218, 501
Wool, O947
Worms, A1508; B910*, C910*, 1616; E498, 500, 1168, 1222*, 1654; F910*; H910*; O351; P675
Wounds, B322; C335, 1106, 1178; D351, 875; E113, 120, 329*, 350, 499, 568, **697**, 700, 993, 1140*, 1168, 1317, 1318, 1351*, 1421*, 1429*; H215* 598*, 1040; V463, 559

Y

Yellow water, E218, 993, **1183**
Young, W, 1727

Z

Zoo, 363, 1727
Zoonoses, 378, 708, 1103, 1139, 1142, 1251, **1290**; see also individual diseases